I congratulate the authors, Dr. Aziz Shaibani, Ms. Abir Zahra, and Dr, Husam Al Sultani for this wonderful book, Coping with Myasthenia Gravis, which will be tremendously helpful for patients and families dealing with this disease. Standard medical textbooks are good for students and clinicians but are not written for patients and family members, because they do not typically deal with how various diseases specifically interrupt their daily lives or advise on coping skills, which often are best given from those that live with the disorders 24/7. This book first describes the history myasthenia gravis, the cause, how it is diagnosed and treated using lay language so that it is easily understandable to all. The second section are short inspirational stories written by 50 patients with myasthenia gravis describing how myasthenia has personally affected their lives, how they have dealt with the disease, fears of what may happen, and side effects of treatments. They give their own practical advice for other patients and families on how to manage by discussing their own personal journeys. Each story is followed by brief comments from an expert clinician. Additionally, the authors cite other helpful resources for patients and families in regard to myasthenia gravis.

In short, I strongly recommend this book. It belongs on the bookshelf of any patient dealing with myasthenia gravis.

Anthony A. Amato, MD
BWH Distinguished Chair in Neurology, Department of Neurology
Chief, Neuromuscular Division
Brigham and Women's Hospital
Professor of Neurology, Harvard Medical School

This is a unique and innovative resource for patients who are trying to navigate the challenges of living with myasthenia gravis. It provides both patient insights and "pearls" as well as expert comment from an experienced clinician, Dr.Shaibani. I would strongly recommend this resource for anyone whose life has been touched with this disease.

Carlayne E. Jackson, MD, FAAN
Professor of Neurology and Otolaryngology
Chief, Neuromuscular section
UT Health San Antonio
President elect, American Academy of Neurology

Dr. Shaibani has another hit on his hands. With his colleagues, Ms. Zahra and Dr. Al Sultani, he has put together a unique book for patients with myasthenia gravis that delivers head-on advice for dealing with the daily trials and tribulations that the disease presents. The book begins with 10 chapters that describe essentially all aspects of the myasthenia, from its history to its treatment. There is even a short chapter on trivia, where the tale of Sleepy, one of Snow White's seven dwarfs, is mentioned.

The second part of the book focuses on patients telling their stories and offering their coping mechanisms. There is advice on everything from swallowing to preparing for surgery, from medications to matters of faith, with additional input provided by Dr. Shaibani. The book is filled with catchy titles, user-friendly information, and whimsical illustrations. Written in a straightforward, easy to digest style,

I believe Dr. Shaibani's latest book will be a valuable resource for patients with myasthenia gravis for years to come. It accomplishes on many levels what we try to do as neuromuscular docs for our patients– explain things so they can be understood and find ways to make their lives easier and more enjoyable.

Gil I. Wolfe, MD
Irvin and Rosemary Smith Professor and Chairman
Dept. of Neurology, Jacobs School of Medicine and Biomedical Sciences
Univ. at Buffalo/SUNY

# COPING WITH Myasthenia Gravis

*Mastering Your Life*

AZIZ SHAIBANI,
A. ZAHRA,
H. AL SULTANI

authorHOUSE®

*AuthorHouse*™
*1663 Liberty Drive*
*Bloomington, IN 47403*
*www.authorhouse.com*
*Phone: 833-262-8899*

*Published by AuthorHouse 02/09/2021*

*ISBN: 978-1-6655-0301-3 (sc)*
*ISBN: 978-1-6655-0375-4 (e)*

*Library of Congress Control Number: 2020923629*

*Print information available on the last page.*

# CONTENTS

# INTRODUCTION

The concept of this book was suggested by several patients who wanted a source of answers for their daily problems in dealing with an unpredictable disease. Accounts in medical textbooks do not reflect the lives of individual patients suffering from and coping with myasthenia gravis symptoms and treatments. Support groups are limited to occasional meetings and sometimes newsletters. There is a need for a source of inspiration and practical advice—for newly diagnosed patients in particular.

There is no book on the market that covers issues that are best addressed by patients who have been through the journey and discovered the best ways to deal with different symptoms, effects, and side effects of medications at different stages and ages. When we participated in *Coping with the Myositis Disease* in the nineties, we never thought that the book would continue to be in demand even twenty years later. Clearly, there is a need for such material.

This book will include self-written stories from fifty patients with myasthenia gravis, describing mostly their experiences fighting the disease and coping with it. Each story will reflect a purely personal, physical, and/or spiritual experience that may be useful to others with the same specific issues. These methods are not validated scientifically and do not essentially reflect universally acceptable methods, but this book is not about scientific exploration or verification. It is about personal experience, which is hardly testable in the laboratory. This represents the humane factor that is missing in the care of patients with myasthenia gravis.

It is hard to describe the feeling of a young lady who faces a new diagnosis, especially when she knows that steroids are the mainstay of treatment despite the horrible side effects, like weight gain and acne. It is hard to match any experience to the uncertainty that patients feel when they run out of medication due to a lack of insurance or affordability, with the possibility of a relapse that may cost them their life. Patients with MG develop a special kind of character that questions every step, and some tend to take the opportunity to change the dose and frequency of their medications on their own. The problem is that symptoms do not return right away; it may take weeks to months, reinforcing the notion that the change in the therapeutic regimen is not responsible. Some patients only learn after they end up in the hospital for relapse and may be intubated.

All these issues will be discussed, supplemented by comments from my twenty-five years of experience treating patients with myasthenia gravis in one of the largest MG clinics in the United States, located in the heart of the largest medical center in the world, Texas Medical Center. I would like to thank my office staff—in particular, Linda Carter, Sandra Villegas, Yeni Villegas, and Karen Dudely—for their support to the patients, who always compliment their attitudes and gestures. I would also like to thank my coauthors, Dr. Husam Al Sultani and Ms. Abir Zahra, whose perspective on medicine as a career was reinforced by writing this book.

I owe this book to its heroes, the patients who took the time to pencil their experiences so that others will benefit, get inspired, and enjoy. I wish them a smooth journey with this chronic but treatable disease.

Aziz Shaibani, MD

# PART ONE

## ABOUT MYASTHENIA GRAVIS

# 1

# THE DISEASE THAT I WOULD CHOOSE

A patient asked me one time, "Out of the ten or so diseases that you treat, which one would you choose if you had to be afflicted with one?"

Without hesitation, I replied, "Myasthenia gravis." It was not because I did not like dealing with ALS, CIDP, diabetic neuropathy, polymyositis, inclusion body myositis, muscular dystrophy, stiff person syndrome, and others. After all, in our tertiary center, we only saw rare and complicated disorders, and I adored every patient regardless of the diagnosis.

I chose MG for two reasons. The first was that it was a fascinating model for autoimmune disease. There are many autoimmune disorders that occur when the immune system reacts against certain body elements that it is supposed to tolerate. But MG is one of the earliest disorders where the role of antibodies in the causation of the disease was demonstrated. Also, their role in the diagnosis cannot be overemphasized.

The second reason is that the disease is treatable, and most patients can return to a normal life. The disease can be funny yet intriguing. It may take a while for MG to be diagnosed by a community physician or even by a neurologist due to the nonspecific nature of the symptoms and the low index of suspicion.

After several visits to the ER, a young patient was diagnosed with a hysterical reaction because no cause was found for her fatigue, blurred vision, shortness of breath, and sometimes swallowing difficulty. All resolved after resting in the ER, and a general inexperienced examination was normal. Only after she was unable to breathe was she admitted, intubated, and then investigated thoroughly so that the diagnosis of MG was made.

The transient and fluctuating nature of the symptoms is due to *fatigability*, a consistent clinical feature of the disease caused by the inability of the muscles to sustain activity due to reduced ability of a chemical called *acetylcholine* to stimulate the muscles to contract because the places (receptors) that the chemical is supposed to occupy are taken up by antibodies formed by the immune system. We do not know why these antibodies are formed. They may be triggered by a viral infection. The disease is not genetic, but family members of an affected person are at a higher risk than the general population.

The most commonly affected muscles are the most delicate ones, because they have more nerve-muscle junctions to control their delicate functions. These include the muscles that are responsible for eye opening, eye movement, swallowing, chewing, and talking. Thus, patients may present with one or both eyelids drooping; trouble swallowing, chewing, and talking; and, sometimes, trouble breathing. All these symptoms are worsened by activity and improved by rest.

Since high temperature is not a good friend of MG, as it slows nerve conduction, these symptoms tend to worsen during the summer, after a hot shower, and when swallowing hot food. A cup of ice cream may improve swallowing, thus allowing the patient to get pills down. Driving during the night becomes hard due to double vision that is worsened by high-intensity light; patching an eye becomes essential to avoid accidents. Chewing becomes so difficult, especially for steak and other foods that require extensive chewing, that some patients learn to support their jaw with their hands during eating. Trouble swallowing is typically more pronounced for liquids, so patients avoid drinking water and become dehydrated, which may worsen their fatigue.

While most patients first experience the disease through double vision or droopy eyelids during activity, the disease will remain confined to the eyes in less than half; this is called *ocular myasthenia gravis*. The rest will experience the spread of symptoms to swallowing, slurred speech, difficulty chewing, and weakened muscles. The good news is that if such a spread (generalization) does not occur in the first two years of the diagnosis, it is very unlikely to happen.

The disease may affect any age, but more so middle-aged women and old men. Fatigability may linger for years before it raises suspicion. Once MG is suspected, the most specific test involves measuring the antibodies (acetylcholine receptor antibodies) against the muscle end of the nerve-muscle junction (postsynaptic membrane). Some patients ask to have these measured to monitor response to treatment. Unfortunately, the function is only diagnostic. The antibodies are not reduced consistently with treatment. They are very specific to myasthenia but occasionally are falsely positive, as in some cases of amyotrophic lateral sclerosis (ALS, commonly referred to as Lou Gehrig's disease). The problem is, they are negative in more than 50 percent of cases of myasthenia, and their negativity should not be used against the diagnosis.

Some MG patients who test negative may have different types of antibodies that should be tested, such as those directed against an enzyme called MuSK and a protein called LRP4. The old edrophonium test is occasionally used today to confirm the diagnosis by injecting a chemical that prevents the breakdown of the enzyme that metabolizes acetylcholine so that the level of acetylcholine increases for a minute or so and the eyelids open. It is not specific and might be associated with side effects.

To confirm the diagnosis, an electrical test called a *repetitive nerve stimulation test* is used. A nerve in the neck or arm is stimulated several times, and the response of the supplied muscle is recorded for undue fatigability. Unfortunately, this test is only positive in 60 percent of cases.

There is a very sensitive test called *single-fiber EMG* that measures the jitter produced by variable responses of muscle fibers to nerve stimulation. It is usually done on a forehead muscle. It can be positive in non-MG patients, such as those with ALS, neuropathy, or a history of trauma to the tested muscle or nerve. However, if it is negative in a weak muscle, MG would be excluded. Considering a positive test as a definitive diagnosis is a common mistake by patients and physicians alike. Computerized axial tomography of the chest is an important part of the diagnostic process to rule out a tumor of the thymus, which occurs in approximately 10 percent of cases.

The most difficult and common scenario is when symptoms are confined to the eyes and all the diagnostic tests are negative. It is important in these cases to rule out brain pathology that may be responsible for the double vision. Also, when slurring of speech is the only finding, it is important to rule out ALS. A medication called *pyridostigmine* is used in mild and ocular cases. It works by increasing the level of acetylcholine in the nerve terminal for four hours after each dose. This medicine sometimes is used to confirm the diagnosis in the mentioned "all negative" cases. However, a positive response is not specific and can only be used along with other parameters and clinical judgment to ascertain the diagnosis.

This medicine can also be used only when needed in established cases of MG. If a patient wants to spend an evening with a friend and enjoy dinner, one or two tablets an hour before eating will help for four hours. Too much of this medicine may cause weakness that can be confused with myasthenic weakness, however. The maximum dose is 540 milligrams per day.

Prednisone is the mainstay of treatment and is often given in a high dose for several months, followed by gradual tapering to the minimum effective maintenance dose that will be continued for at least two years. Side effects are common and can be extensive. However, especially in young patients, it is safer than uncontrolled MG.

Most cases are controllable with prednisone and pyridostigmine. About 20 percent of cases need a steroid-sparing agent because the disease relapses when the prednisone is lowered. There are several agents—such as azathioprine, methotrexate, cyclosporine, and CellCept—that take months to start working, and they are more helpful for long-term control. There are also temporizing remedies, such as intravenous gamma globulin and plasma exchange. These remedies work for four to six weeks and are reserved for severe cases, such as myasthenic crisis (when breathing is compromised) or right before major surgery. However, some patients need them for long-term control of MG due to failure or poor tolerance of the other remedies. In that case, patients will have to take them periodically, ranging from every two weeks to every two months, with or without other treatments.

Eculizumab is the most recent addition to the armamentarium of MG therapy. It is reserved for severe refractory generalized cases that have to be confirmed by positive antibodies. It costs about $500,000 a year and has to be given intravenously every two weeks indefinitely.

Removal of the thymus gland is indicated for patients with a tumor of the thymus gland (thymoma) that is usually benign. However, more than two-thirds of MG patients have an enlargement or reactive increase in the cells of the gland (reactive hyperplasia), usually not visible by a CT scan. Removal of the thymus is indicated in all patients who have MG that has spread beyond the eyes and who are younger than seventy years. Thymectomy reduces the future need for steroids and frequency of crises.

Myasthenia gravis may be exacerbated by psychological or physical stress, such as surgery, pregnancy, childbirth, trauma, and emotions. More importantly, it can be exacerbated by certain medications, such as those used to treat seizures and heart conditions and certain antibiotics. Even eye drops of certain antibiotics can have that effect. Patients should keep an updated list of prohibited medications and should not hesitate to check with their treating physician if they are not sure.

The good news is that the longer the duration of the disease, the more likely it will go into remission. Most complications occur in the first three years after diagnosis.

# 2

# MYASTHENIA GRAVIS

Myasthenia gravis is a rare neuromuscular disease that leads to interruption of communication signals between nerves and muscles, resulting in muscle weakness and muscle fatigue. The Latin name of *myasthenia gravis* translates to "profound muscle weakness," where *myo* means "muscle," *asthenia* means "weakness," and *gravis* means "profound." Although myasthenia gravis is not a common disease, it's considered the most common signaling disease of the neuromuscular junction. There are more than twenty persons in every 100,000 in the US affected by myasthenia gravis. Experts speculate that more people have myasthenia gravis than is known, but because of the difficult diagnosis and its similarity to other neuromuscular diseases, it remains underdiagnosed.

The cause of myasthenia gravis is related to an autoimmune process by which the immune system confuses parts of the body for a target, resulting in tissue damage and loss of function. Normally in a healthy muscle cell, a chemical called acetylcholine[1] binds to a muscle receptor, located in the neuromuscular junction, to produce a muscle contraction. In the case of myasthenia gravis, the body produces antibodies[2] against these muscle receptors, ultimately damaging the receptor. It is not clear why the immune system fails to recognize that these receptors are native, but the most accepted theory is that they have a similar structure to molecules in

---

[1] . Acetylcholine (Ach) is a chemical messenger released from nerve ends to communicate to other cells in the body, such as muscle cells.
[2] . Antibodies are small proteins normally produced to fight viruses and other body invaders.

a gland behind the sternum called the thymus.[3] That is why a tumor of this gland (thymoma[4]) is more common in MG patients. Even without a tumor present, this gland is enlarged in patients with MG and consists of excess cells and lymphoid tissue. This explains the need to remove the thymus in patients with myasthenia gravis.

Patients with MG usually complain of fatigable muscle weakness, meaning strength is lost with repeated or prolonged use. Some muscles are more affected than others, especially muscles involving the eyes, swallowing, speech, and breathing. This explains why patients suffering from MG will experience droopy eyelids, double vision, swallowing difficulties, muscle weakness of the arms and legs, and sometimes breathing problems. MG is diagnosed by the patient's medical history, physical examination, blood tests, electrical stimulation testing, and pharmacological methods. The treatment of MG varies from medications like pyridostigmine to more serious procedures like plasmapheresis.

---

[3] . The thymus is a gland that plays an important role in the immune and endocrine systems.

[4] . A thymoma is a benign tumor arising from the cells of the thymus gland.

# 3

## HISTORY

Although the first description of myasthenia gravis in modern history came in the seventeenth century, no one can be sure how long people have been afflicted by the disease. The symptoms can be confused with those of many other disorders, meaning any disease that causes muscle weakness can be confused with MG, especially if the weakness is fatigable.

The history of medical diseases has been shown to be mixed with superstitious practices and has lacked a scientific approach since antiquity. Nevertheless, Egyptians, Greeks, and Muslims were distinguished for their great advancement in the study of the human body and disease description. Some who contributed to these advancements are philosophers and pioneers of medicine such as Diocles, Avicenna, and Rhazes. They described the nervous system, human anatomy, and some of the most common diseases. They are known as important references for physicians in Western Civilization. Yet myasthenia gravis, a rare disease, has slipped from the grasp of medical history.

The first description of MG dates back to the seventeenth century, when Virginian chroniclers reported that an influential Native American chief known as Opechancanough had muscle weakness that prevented him from walking but could be alleviated by rest. The description went on to explain how Opechancanough had only muscle weakness without prominent issues in his intellect or mental abilities. On the other hand, he exhibited one of the most famous symptoms of MG: "his eyelids were so heavy that he could not see unless they were lifted up by his attendants."[5]

In 1672, the English physician Thomas Willis described a woman who had a "fatiguable weakness"[6] in a Latin text that was ignored until the early 1900s. Willis wrote that the woman "temporarily lost her power of speech and became 'mute as a fish.'"

In the nineteenth century, more reports described cases of MG from German, Polish, and other European physicians like Wilhelm Heinrich Erb, Johann Ignaz Hoppe, and Samuel V. Goldflam. After these numerous reports, MG was described in detail, and its symptoms were well recorded and studied. By the end of the century, the term *myasthenia gravis* was established as the name of the disease.

In 1877, the first case of childhood MG was reported by the English physician Samuel Wilks, while in 1942, the first case report of a newborn with temporary myasthenia gravis was published. A few years later, the term *juvenile myasthenia gravis* was devised to describe the disease in children and adolescents.

In 1949, a doctor by the name of Paul Levin described two siblings with congenital (hereditary) myasthenic syndrome and established congenital myasthenic syndrome as another type of neuromuscular transmission disorder. By the mid-twentieth century, MG was a well-known disease among neurologists and physicians. Eventually, scientists studied the mechanism by which myasthenia gravis affects nerve-muscle communication and the possible causes of the disease. Even before that, there were many attempts to find medications and procedures that would help myasthenic patients and improve their strength.

The first two medications for the treatment of MG were discovered by accident. Before 1929, the main treatment was bedrest and supplements. Most physicians prescribed calcium, minerals, and testicular or thyroid extracts among other ingredients, while others experimented with thymus and thyroid irradiation or radioactive injections. Eventually, adjustments

---

[5] . B. M. Conti-Fine, M. Milani, and H. J. Kaminski, "Myasthenia Gravis: Past, Present, and Future," *Journal of Clinical Investigation* 116, no. 11 (2006): 2843–2854, https://doi.org/10.1172/jci29894.

[6] . Conti-Fine, Milani, and Kaminski, "Myasthenia Gravis: Past, Present, and Future."

were made to this treatment plan due to an accidental finding, as is the case with many discoveries in medicine.

An example of this comes from one of the most influential people who contributed to the treatment of MG while suffering from the disease herself. In the 1930s, Harriet Isabel Edgeworth, a biochemist with MG, was trying to relieve her menstrual cramps by taking ephedrine with aminopyrine (a stimulant and analgesic combination) when she noticed an improvement in her strength. She further studied ephedrine to find out its positive effect as a treatment for MG.

In another coincidence, Mary Broadfoot Walker, a Scottish physician, was talking with a neurologist in her ward when they discussed the similarity between MG and curare poisoning (curare disrupts the nerve-muscle connection) and the antidote for that poison, physostigmine.[7] The young physician injected physostigmine into one of her myasthenic patients and noticed a great improvement in the patient's strength. Since that day, acetylcholinesterase (AChE) inhibitors like pyridostigmine[8] (Mestinon) have been regarded as the first-line treatment for MG.

When steroids were first tried as a treatment in the early 1950s, patients worsened and were sometimes so weak that their respiratory muscles failed. After deserting steroids as a treatment for myasthenia gravis for almost two decades, scientists returned to the use of them, especially when it was found that the worsening was temporary (lasting seven to ten days), with patients undergoing significant improvement afterward. This discovery made steroids more popular in the 1970s and the most important immune suppressant medication in MG treatment to this day.

In the years following this discovery, more immune-lowering drugs were used, particularly after the autoimmune nature of MG was discovered by D. W. Smithers and John Simpson in 1960. This resulted in the improvement of patients' symptoms after depressing their immune system activity.

In 1911, the surgeon Ferdinand Sauerbruch performed a thymus removal surgery (thymectomy) on a patient who happened to have MG. Thymectomy procedures were used to treat increased thyroid hormone in

---

[7] . Physostigmine is a chemical that functions as a cholinesterase inhibitor, meaning it works to increase the concentration of acetylcholine at the necessary sites.

[8] . Pyridostigmine was introduced in 1954.

the body, but Sauerbruch noticed an improvement in MG symptoms rather than in thyroid function. In 1936, Alfred Blalock performed the successful removal of a thymic tumor in a patient with MG. The patient experienced marked and sustained improvement for several years.

Scientists found that 75 percent of patients with MG had an abnormal thymus, and subsequently, a thymectomy was recommended to all patients with generalized MG regardless of the presence of a tumor. This notion was only confirmed scientifically in 2016 through a large clinical trial published in the *New England Journal of Medicine*. In the late 1970s and early 1980s, plasma exchange and intravenous immunoglobulin (IVIG) were introduced as a treatment in myasthenic crisis and patients who didn't improve with other treatment methods. This treatment works to remove or neutralize the antibodies attacking the nerve-muscle connection.

Throughout the years, due to the collective efforts of many scientists and physicians, we have established a firm idea of how myasthenia gravis happens and how to treat it. Thanks to these efforts, patients with myasthenia gravis can almost lead a normal life. Table 1 depicts the timeline of these discoveries.

**Table 1: Timeline of Medical Discoveries in Myasthenia Gravis[9]**

| Date | Event |
| --- | --- |
| 1644 | Earliest description of an American case |
| 1672 | First case described by a physician |
| 1868 | First confirmed case |
| 1877 | First childhood case |
| 1895 | Description of the abnormal neuromuscular junction transmission |
| 1899 | Role of thymic tumor discovered |
| 1911 | First thymectomy in myasthenia gravis |
| 1927 | First familial case |

[9] Afifi, A. K, "Myasthenia Gravis from Thomas Willis to the Present," *Neurosciences (Riyadh)* 10, no. 1 (2005): 3–13.

| 1930 | Use of ephedrine in treatment |
|------|-------------------------------|
| 1934 | Use of physostigmine in treatment |
| 1936 | First thymectomy of a myasthenic patient with thymoma |
| 1942 | First transient neonatal myasthenia case |
| 1950s | Introduction of corticosteroid treatment |
| 1950 | Introduction of Tensilon |
| 1954 | Introduction of pyridostigmine in treatment |
| 1958 | Establishment as an autoimmune disorder |
| 1966 | Steroids reintroduced for treatment |
| 1967 | Azathioprine used for treatment |
| 1976 | Identification of acetylcholine receptor antibody |
| 1976 | Plasma exchange used in myasthenia gravis treatment |
| 1980 | Role of T and B cells defined in the disease mechanism |
| 1984 | IVIG used in myasthenia gravis treatment |
| 1990s | Structure of the acetylcholine receptor defined |

# 4

# EPIDEMIOLOGY

Although MG is considered a rare disease, it is the most common primary disease of neuromuscular transmission. It occurs in all ages, genders, and races, but the distribution of cases is different in each category. In the United States, it is estimated that there are up to 60,000 myasthenia gravis patients, with a rate of fourteen to forty per 100,000. The number of patients has increased since earlier decades, as with most autoimmune disorders.

In the mid-twentieth century, the number of people with myasthenia gravis was three per 100,000 worldwide. That increased to thirty per 100,000 in this decade. Most increments appear to have happened in the elderly. This increase could partly be due to an increase in recognition and awareness of the disease.

MG affects females more than males in a ratio of 3:2, but the ratio varies among age groups. More women have the disease in their third and fourth decades of life, while slightly more men are presented in the sixth and seventh decade. There are more chances for a woman to have MG in midlife, but a man's chances increase in old age. Geography is also a factor in numbers. While it's rare for a child or a teenager to have MG in the Western part of the world (around 10 percent), 30 percent of MG cases in China and Japan are of children below fifteen years old. Race is another factor to consider.

After advances in medicine and medical research, the rate of death and complications from MG has drastically lowered since the 1900s, when almost 100 percent of patients died from MG complications, especially related to respiratory failure because of muscle weakness that affected breathing. In the 2000s, less than 5 percent died as a result of MG. The most noticeable improvement has been the enhancement in breathing support and ventilators.

# 5

# MECHANISM OF MYASTHENIA GRAVIS

In the human body, there are small protein particles called *antibodies*. Antibodies are produced by white blood cells as part of the defense mechanism against viruses or any material not recognized as part of the body, in addition to other functions. Each one of the thousands of antibodies is fit to its complementary receptor like a lock and key to conduct its function in a controlled manner.

Sometimes, for reasons that are yet unknown, the immune system produces antibodies against its own elements, such as muscles. This type of disease is called an *autoimmune disorder*. Myasthenia gravis in most cases happens in the same way, with antibodies attacking their own nerve-muscle junction and specifically blocking the acetylcholine receptors, thereby preventing contraction of the muscle fiber.

To understand the process of nerve-muscle transmission, imagine two plates opposed to each other and separated by a small space. One plate represents the nerve ending while the other is the muscle ending. When an electrical signal reaches the nerve ending, a chemical material (acetylcholine) is released, crosses, and reaches the muscle plate, where it connects to receptors fitted for its structure. After acetylcholine connects the receptors, the muscle is activated and contraction occurs. In MG, antibodies against these receptors are the cause of a signal interruption and stop the muscles from contracting—hence the characteristic weakness. If enough acetylcholine presents to the receptors, the muscle should contract, but when there are fewer receptors because of autoantibodies, there will not be enough receptors to stimulate a reaction.

Scientists have studied MG painstakingly for decades to understand its underlying process. In numerous studies, the thymus gland was a prime suspect, with 10 percent of MG patients having a thymoma (benign tumor of the thymus), while inversely, up to 50 percent of patients with thymoma will have MG. The thymus is a small gland that lies in the chest and is considered a major organ in the production of T-lymphocytes cells (white blood cells that help in defense and immunity). In many MG patients, the thymus is overactive, and sometimes its cells undergo transformation to become a thymoma. The relation between a malfunctioning thymus and MG is supported by the favorable effect of thymectomy on a myasthenic patient.

More than one type of antibody has been found to cause the disease process. The most common are antibodies against acetylcholine receptors (anti-AChR antibodies) and antibodies against MuSK (anti-MuSK antibodies). MuSK, or muscle-specific kinase, is a protein in the space between nerve and muscle that plays a major role in signal transmission. Although the two antibodies are the most commonly found in myasthenia gravis patients, other antibodies can also be responsible for the disease process but are less commonly implicated. A small percentage of MG cases are not associated with any known antibodies. This type is known as *seronegative myasthenia gravis*, meaning the blood test that checks for MG antibodies will yield negative results for the testable MG-related antibodies.

In general, MG pathology is related to autoantibodies against the components of nerve-muscle connection, either by causing the destruction of acetylcholine receptors in the muscle end or by directly blocking the attachment of acetylcholine to these receptors. Another factor that causes blocking of the nerve-muscle signal are protein particles called *complement factors*. Complements are part of the defense mechanism against foreign offenders, and like antibodies, they can turn against the body and cause damage that manifests as a disease.

Unlike MG, congenital myasthenic syndromes are negative for the antibodies and have a genetic cause that can usually be identified by genetic testing. Patients rarely have both the autoimmune and hereditary version of the disease.

# 6

## Clinical Features

The most notable feature of myasthenia gravis is the muscle weakness experienced as the first sign of the disease. However, it is a particular type of muscle weakness that is said to be fluctuating. This means the weakness is not always present or does not stay at the same intensity throughout the day.

Because of the way MG affects individuals, muscle weakness increases when that specific muscle is used and improves after rest to allow the transmission chemicals that were depleted to build up again in the junction between a muscle and a nerve. Of course, in chronic and poorly treated cases, the weakness may not subside with rest, although this is uncommon today.

Another feature of muscle weakness is the specific muscle groups affected. The most common are the muscles of the eyes and eyelid movement. This group of muscles is responsible for moving the eyes in all directions in a very coordinated fashion to create very close images by both eyes. When one or more of the six muscles in each eye are affected, there will be a larger discrepancy between the images from both eyes, and therefore diplopia. The delicate muscles in the eyelids are often affected in MG and droop or fatigue easily, leading to ptosis.

The other muscle groups commonly affected include the following:

- **Swallowing**—When MG affects the muscles involved in swallowing, it can lead to choking on liquids more often than solids.
- **Facial**—Other muscles of the face and throat will result in speech difficulties, facial expression abnormality, and chewing tiredness.
- **Arms, legs, neck**—Weakness of the muscles in the arms, legs, or neck will lead to impairment of the functions of limbs, such walking, standing up, or holding things with the arms as well as head movement.
- **Breathing**—The most serious and dangerous muscle group to be affected are the breathing muscles; these include the diaphragm, which is a domelike muscle that helps the lungs to inhale and exhale, and the outside muscles that control the widening and narrowing of the chest to allow air movement in and out of the lungs. The weakness of the breathing muscles will lead to respiratory compromise, and sometimes the patient will need breathing assistance and hospitalization.

The first symptoms developed in MG patients can vary, but in most instances, the eye muscles are the first to be affected, which can cause problems with one or both eyes. The muscles of the jaws, throat, and face often follow. It is rare to have the breathing muscles as the first to be affected in MG; rather, it occurs as a sign that the disease is worsening and may happen a few years after the first symptoms have developed.

The progression of MG varies from person to person. The disease may start as mildly as simple double vision or as severely as generalized muscle weakness. In most cases, there are predictable factors that may worsen symptoms, such as stress, heat, infection, medications, or pregnancy.

A mother with MG can deliver a baby with MG symptoms that may last for the first several weeks, but this course tends to be temporary. It is called *infantile myasthenia gravis.*

The most serious complication of MG is an exacerbation of symptoms that sometimes leads to a myasthenic crisis. A *myasthenic crisis* is defined as an abrupt increase in MG symptoms, such as increased muscle weakness, especially with the muscles involved in breathing. This could necessitate breathing assistance and artificial ventilation.[10] Usually, a myasthenic crisis is triggered by infections, stress, surgery, and drugs, although sometimes the cause cannot be identified. When MG patients experience a crisis, they need emergency identification and treatment. In the past, a myasthenic crisis was a deadly complication, but with advanced medicine and care, the death rate has fallen significantly to below 5 percent.

---

[10] . An artificial machine that pumps air in the lungs when breathing becomes a problem

# 7

## CLASSIFICATION

Myasthenia gravis can be classified according to the symptoms or causative antibodies. About 60 percent of MG cases are due to anti-ACh receptor antibodies. About 50 percent of the negative ones are caused by MuSK antibodies. Other rare antibodies have been identified, like LRP4 and agrin antibodies, which have recently become available for testing. Still, about 20 percent of cases are seronegative, although their sera[11] are pathogenic to animals.

Symptomatically, there are two types of myasthenia gravis: ocular and generalized. *Ocular* means related to the eyes. In ocular MG, the earliest symptoms arise from weakness in the eyes and eyelid muscles, resulting in double vision and drooped eyelids (ptosis). About 50 percent of cases start as ocular, and half of those will become generalized. About 20 percent start as bulbar (swallowing, speech, and or chewing fatigability), and 10 percent start in the extremities.

When ocular MG stays confined to the eye muscles for more than two years, it's likely to stay that way. The term *generalized myasthenia gravis* is used to describe the case when the disease has spread beyond the eye muscles. It is rare that shortness of breath is the presenting symptom.

Furthermore, MG can be divided into two categories when the age of onset is considered: early onset and late onset. There has been a debate over the age at which MG should be considered early or late onset. Lately, it has been determined that fifty years old is the cutoff value. Early onset

---

[11] . Plural form of *serum*

MG is the classic presentation of the disease, and studies have found gender differences, with females three times more likely to have early onset MG than males.

Early onset MG has specific features that differentiate it. For example, it is more aggressive and resistant to treatment. The thymus is enlarged, and it's associated with other autoimmune diseases like thyroid diseases and Lupus. Since the first cases of MG were reported, early onset incidence has been stable, while late onset incidence has increased, resulting in a skewed ratio of early to late onset.

Males have almost equal chances to have late onset MG as females. In this type, MG has a milder course and better response to treatment. The thymus is atrophied.[12] Nevertheless, in this age category, MG is less likely to go into remission, and the death rate is higher compared to other diseases people have at that age.

In 10 to 15 percent of MG cases, a tumor of the thymus is present, which is called a *thymoma*. A thymoma is usually a benign tumor, but it can be very aggressive locally. Although it does not spread like cancer, it produces a large number of cells that in turn produce wide ranges of autoantibodies, some of which can cause MG. Thymoma-related MG occurs in people age forty to sixty and tends to be more severe than other types.

Approximately 6 percent of those with MG develop anti-MuSK antibodies while lacking other antibodies known to be found in MG patients (rarely does a patient have both types of antibodies). Anti-MuSK antibodies related to MG have distinctive geography among other types; for unknown reasons, they are more common in Mediterranean regions and similar latitudes in Asia and North America, but the rate decreases going north. Also, the rate among African Americans is higher than for the white population. In this category, MG is generalized—more severely affecting the muscles involved in swallowing, the face, and breathing—and more resistant to treatment.

A minority of MG cases fall into another type where no MG-related antibodies can be found. This type has a wide range of symptoms but, due to its rarity, is not well studied.

Although there is no widely accepted classification for MG among all

---

12 . The thymus is usually atrophied or diminished in size after age sixty.

specialists, the Myasthenia Gravis Foundation of America (MGFA) has adopted a clinical classification for physicians that divides MG into five classes and more subclasses. The following is a highlight of these classes:[13]

- **class 1**—weakness of eye muscles and/or eyelid muscles with normal strength of the other muscle groups
- **class 2**—mild (slight) weakness of muscle groups other than eye and eyelid muscles (regardless of the involvement of the latter muscles)
- **class 3**—moderate (medium) weakness of muscle groups other than eye and eyelid muscles (regardless of the involvement of the latter muscles)
- **class 4**—severe (serious) weakness of muscle groups other than eye and eyelid muscles (regardless of the involvement of the latter muscles)
- **class 5**—intubation (inserting breathing tube) with or without mechanical breathing assistance

These classes can help healthcare professionals to assess MG severity and help guide treatment.

---

[13] . A. Jaretzki 3rd, R. J. Barohn, R. M. Ernstoff, et. al., "Myasthenia Gravis: Recommendations for Clinical Research Standards: Task Force of the Medical Scientific Advisory Board of the Myasthenia Gravis Foundation of America," *Ann Thorac Surg.* 70, no. 1 (2000): 327–334, https://doi.org/10.1016/s0003-4975(00)01595-2.

# 8

## Diagnosis

A physician will suspect myasthenia gravis when a patient presents with muscle weakness, especially a kind of weakness that worsens after using the muscle and improves after rest. As with all illnesses, the first step in diagnosis is history-taking and physical examination. After listening to the patient's subjective take on events and performing a preliminary examination, the physician will have an idea of what to suspect and construct a mental list of the diseases to investigate.

The second step involves testing for suspected diseases to confirm one disease or rule out another.[14] Some tests are simple blood draws or electrical stimulation; others may include surgeries like a biopsy. In the case of MG, after history-taking and examination, a series of tests are required to establish the diagnosis of myasthenia gravis. The first is a blood test to look for antibodies associated with MG, specifically anti-AchR and anti-MuSK antibodies. Testing of antibodies in a patient's blood is simple and is available in most labs.

About 80 percent of generalized MG cases have anti-AChR in their blood, and this test is rarely positive in patients without MG, such as in some cases of thymoma and ALS; this makes the test very specific for

---

[14] . Amyotrophic lateral sclerosis (ALS), Lambert-Eaton myasthenic syndrome, and congenital myasthenic syndromes are examples of diseases similar to MG.

MG.[15] However, it is not very sensitive, as it is negative in 40 percent of ocular MG and 20 percent of generalized MG.

If the blood test was negative for antibodies, some physicians use a pharmaceutical test called edrophonium (Tensilon), in which a chemical called edrophonium is injected into the bloodstream and a patient's response is obtained. Edrophonium works like pyridostigmine by increasing acetylcholine availability in the nerve-muscle connection, so an improvement of muscle weakness means a positive test. Although Tensilon is fast, it is less commonly used nowadays because of poor specificity, side effects, and poor reliability.

Another type of testing is electrophysiological tests. There are two tests involved here: repetitive nerve stimulation and single-fiber electromyography. In repetitive nerve stimulation, a nerve is stimulated repeatedly by a stimulator, and the muscle contraction response is recorded. After a few successive signals are introduced and recorded, a trained physician can determine whether the drop in response is consistent with MG. This is only positive in 60 percent of cases, and more than one nerve needs to be tested. In single-fiber electromyography, a very thin needle is inserted into a muscle to study the electrical signal in two muscle fibers that belong to the same motor unit.[16]

Both tests require a trained specialist and equipment. Single-fiber electromyography is 99 percent sensitive, but it can be positive in conditions that also have an interruption in the nerve signal to the muscle, such as ALS, facial palsy, and trauma.

As mentioned before, myasthenia gravis is associated with an abnormal thymus. In this case, imaging is needed to see if the thymus gland is enlarged or has a tumor. Mostly, a CT scan with contrast injection is used, but sometimes an MRI is needed if a tumor is suspected and is spreading to other organs.

---

[15] . Specificity in testing means the test's ability to correctly designate a person who does not have a disease as negative. If a test is considered to have high specificity, there will be very few false positives.

[16] . Each muscle fiber measures less than a hundred micrometers, where a micrometer is one millionth of a meter.

# 9

# TREATMENT

Myasthenia gravis is a chronic and usually lifelong disease, but its management is simple in most cases. With advancements in medicine every few years, we have witnessed the emergence of a new drug.

To understand MG treatments, it's essential to understand the mechanism behind the disease and how it functions. Myasthenia gravis is both a neuromuscular and an autoimmune disease in association with an abnormal thymus gland, so treatments target one or more of these mechanisms.

The first line of treatment is drugs prescribed to treat symptoms of muscle weakness caused by MG. These drugs are called *acetylcholinesterase inhibitors* (AChE-I), and they make acetylcholine more available by preventing (inhibiting) the enzyme responsible for its removal from the nerve-muscle connection. Many drugs from this family are being used, but the most common is pyridostigmine. Every medicine has side effects; the most common for AChE-I are stomach cramps, sweating, diarrhea, salivation, and muscle cramps. The effects are usually short-lived, and the drug does not change the natural history of the disease, so it is reserved for mild cases.

In the second step of the treatment plan for MG, physicians use drugs that suppress immunity and reduce the production of antibodies called *immunosuppressants*. These drugs are used when the first line of treatment fails to improve the weakness. These are drugs that modify the course of the disease. Steroids are widely used in the treatment plan for MG as well as other autoimmune diseases; of these, prednisone is the usual drug of choice. Prednisone has been very effective with MG but can reduce bone density (osteoporosis), increase blood pressure, and cause weight gain, stomach ulcers, fluid retention, and infections. Therefore, steroids require close monitoring of patients and careful dose titration. Many immunosuppressive medications are available if steroids fail or are not tolerated.

Long-term immunosuppressive drugs can be used to spare patients from steroids' unpleasant side effects. An example of a steroid-sparing agent is azathioprine, a drug that inhibits DNA and RNA production and thus affects the growth of cells responsible for the function of antibodies. Azathioprine is a preferable drug with tolerable side effects, such as stomach upset, bowel motion disturbances, and flulike symptoms—although it takes more than six months to observe its effects on MG symptoms. Other drugs that work in a similar manner as azathioprine are mycophenolate mofetil, cyclosporin, cyclophosphamide, methotrexate, and others. These drugs increase the risk of cancer if used for many years.

A more recent line of drugs used in myasthenia gravis, called monoclonal antibodies or biologics, is a type of antibody that targets certain elements in the immunity process of the body. Some examples are rituximab, eculizumab, and belimumab. These drugs are expensive, and most of them are injected or infused through the vein. Most of them are new and still under study, but physicians use them as an alternative to first- and second-line medications. Most of the side effects here are related to lower immunity and IV administration issues.

Since the thymus is involved in the MG mechanism, removal of the thymus (thymectomy) has become a part of the treatment for generalized MG in those under the age of sixty-five. Those suffering from MG caused by anti-MuSK have not seen better results after a thymectomy. A thymectomy is better performed early in the disease and can provide increased chances of remission (that is, no more or minimal symptoms). A thymectomy is done either by traditional surgery—with an incision and opening of the chest wall—or with a tiny camera introduced through a small hole in the chest (thoracoscopy). A thymectomy is more effective if done within five years of the diagnosis and is indicated in cases of thymoma regardless of age and type of symptoms.

Occasionally, those suffering from MG can go through a myasthenic crisis. This is when a sudden increase in symptoms can put a patient's health at risk. In this case, a faster method of treatment is needed to help suppress immunity and hold off antibody action. Plasma exchange and intravenous immunoglobulin (IVIG) are the two most commonly used methods to address the increased severity of the autoimmune nature of MG.

Plasma exchange is simply cleansing the blood of autoantibodies using an external machine. In this process, blood is drawn from the patient, put through a special machine that removes antibodies, then transfused back into the same patient without the harmful proteins. IVIG, in contrast, is a type of prepared antibody solution that is infused to the bloodstream through an intravenous catheter. The mechanism of IVIG is complex and involves immunity manipulation through its effect on the cells and proteins of the human immune system. It works to neutralize bad antibodies.

Plasma exchange and IVIG are almost equally effective methods of treating MG exacerbation, but the former is usually only available in large institutions, while IVIG can be given at any infusion center or even in the patient's home. Both work for a few weeks, during which the patient has to use other long-term measures like steroids and chemotherapy. However, on rare occasions, they become the only and long-term mode of treatment. Plasma exchange can cause low blood pressure and allergic reactions, while IVIG has more tolerable side effects consisting of headaches, allergies, and renal impairments, especially in diabetics. The treating physician is the one to decide which is indicated.

Although pregnancy in MG is managed differently, the disease itself can cause minor complications in its mild and moderate status. Attention is directed toward treatments of MG and their side effects. Pyridostigmine and the like do not pose a threat to the baby's health but are to be avoided because they can cause contractions of the uterus. Steroids such as prednisone are the first choice for treatment and are closely monitored for side effects.

Other immunosuppressive medications are to be avoided in pregnancy, especially during the first trimester, due to their effect on the development of the embryo. The involvement of high-risk obstetricians is recommended because severe fatigue during labor may necessitate a cesarean section. After delivery, the baby should be examined for transient myasthenia gravis symptoms, since MG-related antibodies can be transferred from mother to child. Poor suckling or breathing or weak crying would be the signs to look for.

Finally, MG patients usually need close follow-ups. Infections are to be treated promptly, and vaccinations need to be administrated on schedule, especially the seasonal flu vaccination, in order to prevent infections. A high risk of breathing muscle involvement warrants attention to lung function to strengthen respiration. Furthermore, side effects from medications, particularly steroids, need to be monitored and corrected. Some examples include decreased bone density and obesity. Patients are usually prescribed calcium and vitamin D for their bones and advised to make lifestyle changes to prevent diabetes and high blood pressure.

Drugs to be avoided or monitored in MG include those on the chart below.[17]

| Drug | Usage | Use in Myasthenia Gravis |
|------|-------|--------------------------|
| telithromycin | antibiotic for pneumonia. | avoid |
| fluoroquinolones antibiotics (e.g., ciprofloxacin, moxifloxacin) | commonly prescribed antibiotics | use with caution |
| botulinum toxin | cosmetic and muscle paralysis | avoid |
| D-penicillamine | used for Wilson disease and rarely for rheumatoid arthritis | strongly associated with causing MG; avoid |
| quinine | occasionally used for leg cramps | prohibited in the US except for malaria |
| magnesium | high blood pressure during late pregnancy or for low blood magnesium | use only if absolutely necessary and observe for worsening |

---

[17] . Source: Myasthenia Gravis Foundation of America

| macrolide antibiotics (e.g. erythromycin, azithromycin) | commonly prescribed antibiotics for bacterial infections | may worsen MG; use with caution |
|---|---|---|
| aminoglycoside antibiotics (e.g. gentamycin, neomycin) | bacterial infections | may worsen MG; use with caution |
| procainamide | irregular heart rhythm | may worsen MG; use with caution |
| desferrioxamine | hemochromatosis disease | may worsen MG; use with caution |
| beta-blockers (e.g. propranolol, metoprolol) | commonly prescribed for high blood pressure, heart disease, and migraine | may worsen MG; use with caution |
| contrast agents | imaging studies | use cautiously and observe for worsening |
| chloroquine (Aralen) | malaria and amoeba infections | may worsen or precipitate MG; use with caution |
| hydroxychloroquine (plaquenil) | malaria, rheumatoid arthritis, and lupus | may worsen or precipitate MG; use with caution |
| immune checkpoint inhibitors (e.g. pembrolizumab, nivolumab) | certain kinds of cancer | may worsen or precipitate MG; use with caution |

# 10

## TRIVIA

It was rumored that Sleepy, a character from the Disney animated movie *Snow White and the Seven Dwarfs*, was inspired by a friend of Walt Disney who had myasthenia gravis.

- The president of the Philippines, Rodrigo Duterte, has myasthenia gravis. On one occasion, he said, "One of my eyes is smaller. It roams on its own." He later disclosed his disease "That's myasthenia gravis. It's a nerve malfunction. I got it from my grandfather."[18]
- After Bollywood's famous Indian actor Amitabh Bachchan suffered an accident and consequently had surgery in 1982, he was diagnosed with myasthenia gravis, which later went into remission.
- The American actor Karl Malden had myasthenia gravis. He once said, "Everybody who knows me knows that I have myasthenia gravis. The doctors don't know how to cure it."[19]
- Until 1930, patients with myasthenia gravis were treated by giving adrenal gland, thymus, ovarian, and testicular extractions along with radioactive thorium injections and thyroid or thymus irradiation.

---

[18] . "Philippines Leader Rodrigo Duterte Says He Has Autoimmune Disease," *The Guardian*, October 7, 2019, https://www.theguardian.com/world/2019/oct/07/philippines-leader-rodrigo-duterte-autoimmune-disease-myasthenia-gravis.

[19] . J. Roberts, "Company Man," *Variety*, February 17, 2004, https://variety.com/2004/film/awards/company-man-1117900232/.

- Although most cases of myasthenia gravis are not hereditary, there is some type of association between certain types of proteins called HLA and myasthenia gravis, so several members of the same family can have myasthenia gravis.

# Helpful Resources

Myasthenia Gravis Foundation of America
https://myasthenia.org/

Myasthenia Gravis Association
http://www.mgakc.org/

Conquer Myasthenia Gravis
https://www.myastheniagravis.org/

Mayo Clinic
https://www.mayoclinic.org/diseases-conditions/myasthenia-gravis/symptoms-causes/syc-20352036

Muscular Dystrophy Association
https://www.mda.org/disease/myasthenia-gravis

National Organization for Rare Disorders
https://rarediseases.org/rare-diseases/myasthenia-gravis/

National Institute of Neurological Disorder and Stroke
https://www.ninds.nih.gov/disorders/patient-caregiver-education/fact-sheets/myasthenia-gravis-fact-sheet

European Myasthenia Gravis Association
https://www.efna.net/members/eumga/

*Aziz Shaibani, A. Zahra, H. Al Sultani*

Myasthenia Alliance Australia
https://myastheniaallianceaustralia.com.au/

The Australian Myasthenic Association in NSW
https://www.myasthenia.org.au/

# REFERENCE

Afifi, A. K. "Myasthenia Gravis from Thomas Willis to the Present." *Neurosciences (Riyadh)* 10, no. 1 (2005): 3–13.

Carr, A. S., C. R. Cardwell, P. O. McCarron, et. al. "A Systematic Review of Population Based Epidemiological Studies in Myasthenia Gravis." *BMC Neurol* 10, no. 46 (2010).

"Celebs Who've Fought Serious Illnesses and Inspired Us to Stay Strong." *The Economic Times*, https://economictimes.indiatimes.com/magazines/panache/celebrities-who-have-fought-serious-illnesses-and-inspired-us-to-stay-strong/amitabh-bachchan/slideshow/64942649.cms.

Conti-Fine, B. M., M. Milani, and H. J. Kaminski. "Myasthenia Gravis: Past, Present, and Future." *Journal of Clinical Investigation* 116, no. 11 (2006): 2843–2854. https://doi.org/10.1172/jci29894.

Hughes, T. "The Early History of Myasthenia Gravis." *Neuromuscular Disorders* 15, no. 12 (2005): 878-886. https://doi.org/10.1016/j.nmd.2005.08.007.

Jaretzki, A. 3rd, R. J. Barohn, R. M. Ernstoff, et. al. "Myasthenia Gravis: Recommendations for Clinical Research Standards: Task Force of the Medical Scientific Advisory Board of the Myasthenia Gravis Foundation of America, *Ann Thorac Surg.* 70, no. 1 (2000): 327–334. https://doi.org/10.1016/s0003-4975(00)01595-2.

Keesey, J. "Myasthenia Gravis." *Archives of Neurology* 55, no. 5 (1998): 745. https://doi.org/10.1001/archneur.55.5.745.

Kennedy, F. S., and F. P. Moersch. "Myasthenia Gravis: A Clinical Review of Eighty-Seven Cases Observed between 1915 and the Early Part of 1932." *Can Med Assoc J.* 37, no. 3 (1937): 216–223.

Lisak, R. P. *Handbook of Myasthenia Gravis and Myasthenic Syndromes.* New York: Marcel Dekker, 1994.

Marsteller, H. B. "The First American Case of Myasthenia Gravis." *Arch Neurol* 45, no. 2 (1988): 185–187. https://doi.org/10.1001/archneur.1988.00520260073024.

"Myasthenia Gravis." Mayo Clinic. Published May 23, 2019. https://www.mayoclinic.org/diseases-conditions/myasthenia-gravis/symptoms-causes/syc-20352036.

"Myasthenia Gravis." NORD (National Organization for Rare Disorders). Published November 1, 2019. https://rarediseases.org/rare-diseases/myasthenia-gravis/.

"Philippines Leader Rodrigo Duterte Says He Has Autoimmune Disease." *The Guardian*, October 7, 2019, https://www.theguardian.com/world/2019/oct/07/philippines-leader-rodrigo-duterte-autoimmune-disease-myasthenia-gravis.

Roberts, J. "Company Man," *Variety*, February 17, 2004, https://variety.com/2004/film/awards/company-man-1117900232/.

Sanders, D. B., G. I. Wolfe, M. Benatar, et. al. "International Consensus Guidance for Management of Myasthenia Gravis." *Neurology* 87, no. 4 (2016): 419–425. https://doi.org/10.1212/wnl.0000000000002790.

Trouth, A. J., A. Dabi, N. Solieman, M. Kurukumbi, and J. Kalyanam. "Myasthenia Gravis: a Review." *Autoimmune Diseases* 874680 (2012). https://doi.org/10.1155/2012/874680.

Video Atlas of neuromuscular disorders. Aziz Shaibani. Oxford University press. 2018, second edition.

# PART TWO
## PATIENTS TELL THEIR STORIES

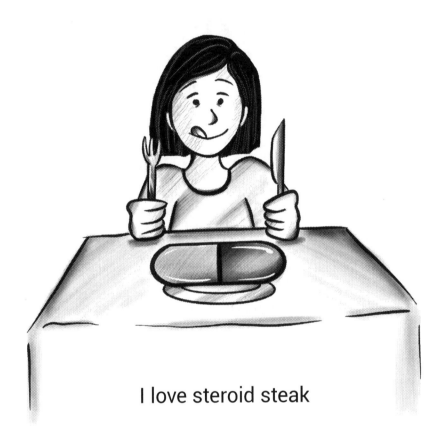

I love steroid steak

# Case #1

## HAPPY SWALLOWING

I found out it is important to not get liquid or food into my lungs. These are my tips for how to deal with swallowing difficulties.

Though it is not acceptable socially, bow your head to the front. This helps separate the food in your mouth from the air you are breathing. When you are starting to eat and you do not want to swallow, move the food from the right side of your mouth to the left and back again while chewing. Also, with the mouth full of well-chewed food, bring the food from your throat back into your mouth. Now add water to your mouth, with your head bowed. Swallow some of the water, then continue chewing. When the swallowing stops, clear your throat back into your mouth. Add water and swallow some of the water; continue chewing. Remember to keep your head bowed as much as possible. Adding the water allows you to start swallowing.

If someone asks you a question, hold your hand up in the wait position until your mouth and throat are clear. Do not try to talk until your mouth and throat are clear. A lot less coughing that way.

Do not use liquids thicker than milk to start swallowing. When you are going to throw up, have an extra plate, bowl, or container available. Coughing, coughing, and coughing—always so much coughing. Swallow water and start with solids again.

How do I get this gel cap to go more than halfway down my throat? Place the capsule on the back of the tongue. Put a good amount of water in your mouth. Move the water to the back of the tongue and swallow big!

Remember to keep your head bowed. Large dry pills like multivitamins, I chew and eat food to kill the taste.

Happy swallowing.

> *"Do not use liquids thicker than milk to start swallowing."*

**Expert Comment:**

Swallowing difficulty is one of the most common and serious manifestations of MG. It is caused by weakness of the pharyngeal muscles, and it is more pronounced for liquids. That is why patients avoid water and stick to semiliquid food.

Good chewing may help prepare the bolus for swallowing, but chewing is often impaired as well, leading to poorly prepared food for swallowing. Chin-tucking (keeping the head bowed) is a useful trick to keep the air pipe closed and the food pipe open. Lack of coordination of the opening of these two pipes leads to aspiration when food goes to the trachea instead of the esophagus and sometimes causes aspiration pneumonia.

Frequent throat-clearing is the earliest symptom of impaired swallowing due to accumulation of saliva. On average, a human produces 1.5 liters of saliva a day, but we never feel it because of the intact constant swallowing mechanism. When this is impaired, saliva accumulates. At night, people can choke on their own saliva.

Choking is the second phase of swallowing impairment and may lead to lack of adequate feeding and dehydration. The variant of MG that is caused by MUSK antibodies is notorious in causing trouble swallowing and even shrinkage of the pharyngeal muscles and weakness of the tongue. Swallowing problems lead to inability to take oral medications, which in turn leads to further worsening of the symptoms.

Patients with mild swallowing difficulty may benefit from taking pyridostigmine an hour before meals. Some patients put the pill in a cube full of Jell-O to facilitate swallowing. Impairment of swallowing correlates with impairment of speech and chewing. These are all called *bulbar functions*.

> *"Some patients put their pill in a cube
> full of Jell-O to facilitate swallowing."*

Never lose hope

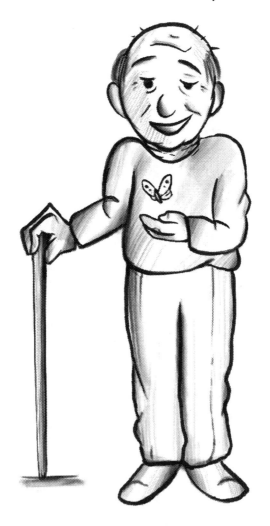

# Case #2

## LIFE IS GREAT

At the age of seventy-two, my earliest symptoms, in October 2012, were a drooping eyelid in my left eye and double vision. I initially went to my eye doctor, and after a thorough examination, he referred me to a neurologist specializing in myasthenia gravis. This specialist performed several tests and finally diagnosed me with MG, then immediately proceeded to put me on a treatment plan in January 2013. After initially starting me on a drug that helped for a couple of months, he eventually, after the original symptoms returned, prescribed prednisone 80 mg a day, plus Pepcid AC 20 mg, calcium 1,000 IU, vitamin D3 1,000 IU, and a daily megavitamin (Centrum). The side effects were sleeplessness and tremendous swelling of the face, weight gain, and irritability.

After what seemed like a prolonged period, much to my delight, my doctor began to gradually lower my dose of prednisone. Everything seemed to be progressing well until, one day in early autumn a few years later, I decided to get a flu shot and a pneumonia shot at the same time. Within a day or two, all the old symptoms came back, and the results were devastating.

Not only did I have to go back to 80 mg a day of prednisone, but I also lost control of my neck and head. I had to lie down every thirty minutes or so because I could not hold up my head. I began to wear a neck brace, and, as a chief accounting officer for a local corporation, I had to begin working from home. I became very depressed thinking this was the beginning of the end and that I was in a downward spiral that would eventually proceed down my body until I would become totally debilitated.

However, very gradually, thanks to my treatment, I began to improve.

My neck became stronger, and I was able to hold up my head without any support. I was finally able to return to work, and after quite a prolonged period, my doctor finally began to lower my prednisone and introduced another complementary drug, azathioprine 50 mg three times a day, in the hopes that he would be able to continue reducing the dose of prednisone. The results have been more than I had hoped for. I have been able to continue working full time. My prednisone dose has now been gradually reduced to 15 mg every other day.

I used to be full of energy in my youth, and much to my surprise, it has returned a great deal. I am once again quite active and enjoying life again to the fullest. I exercise weekly, have a massage every week, will be entertaining my family and friends at Christmas time as always, and am planning a fifteen-day trip to Europe in the spring by myself.

The biggest lesson I have learned is not to take any prescription or get any shots without the full approval of the doctor who is monitoring your MG. My faith in my doctor and his knowledge and expertise is beyond comparison. I feel that he has given me back my life once again, and my gratitude is boundless. Now, in my eightieth year, I can honestly say life is great, thanks to him.

> *"My faith in my doctor and his knowledge and expertise is beyond comparison."*

**Expert Comment:**

While steroids are usually enough to induce remission, sometimes the disease relapses when prednisone is tapered and before a safe maintenance dose of 10 to 20 mg every other day is reached. In these cases, adding a steroid-sparing agent like azathioprine would be useful. However, it will take several months before it starts working, during which the patient will stay on a high dose of prednisone, which increases the risk of side effects.

The medication is usually well tolerated. Rarely, patients develop an immediate reaction that consists of severe dizziness, stomach upset, and diarrhea. Long-term side effects are rare but can be serious, like a severe drop in white cell count that would make the patient vulnerable to infection. For that reason, a monthly checking of the white cell count is advised and may be needed more frequently at the start. Mild liver toxicity is also reported, for which the blood level of some liver enzymes is checked monthly.

There is no consensus as to how long azathioprine use should continue. Most experts advocate trying every two years to gradually stop it and see if the disease comes back. Azathioprine may interact with some medications—especially allopurinol, which is used for gout—because they compete on the same enzymes, leading to increased toxicity. There is a concern that using azathioprine for years may increase the risk of malignancy.

The other important question that this story raises is the relationship between vaccinations and exacerbation of MG. Patients often call during vaccination sessions inquiring about this. There is no evidence that any of the vaccinations participate in MG exacerbation. Unless a specific patient has a documented allergy or reaction to any vaccination, there is no problem with vaccinations in this regard.

During the fall, the risk of exacerbation is high due to the prevalence of the flu. Vaccination will reduce that risk. Patients with MG are prone to more complications from pneumonia, influenza, COVID19, and other infections due to the risk of exacerbation, the risk of respiratory compromise, and the risk associated with immunosuppression from medications like steroids and azathioprine. Therefore, they are advised to stay away from sick children and large crowds.

> *"Vaccination against the flu and COVID19 are recommended to patients with MG."*

Everything will be fine, son

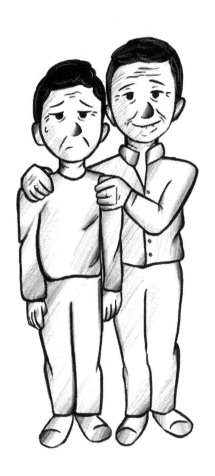

# Case #3

## ACCEPT, TRUST, AND COMMUNICATE

"Depression is a common complication of long-
term steroid therapy... Antidepressants are
helpful and do not exacerbate MG."

I am a sixty-six-year-old white male and have had myasthenia gravis for almost five years. My earliest symptoms were a drooping in my right eyelid and slightly slurred speech. Normally, the symptoms appeared toward the end of the day or when I was stressed or upset.

My first thought when the symptoms appeared was, *I have had a mild stroke.* So, I scheduled an appointment with my primary-care physician to begin the testing process to identify my problem. I had open-heart surgery in 1998 and thought I should see my cardiologist first to be sure it was not heart-related. Then I saw a pulmonary doctor to ensure my lungs were okay. Both checked out fine.

At the advice of my brother, I was tested by a neurologist for MG. You may ask, where did that come from and why? Well, my dad had MG, and we had a common symptom: the drooping eyelid. MG is not supposed to be hereditary, but in my case, it was. Lucky me, right?

After my initial diagnosis of MG, I was referred to a doctor who specializes in it. Within a month, the diagnosis of MG was confirmed by the specialist. My first reaction to the diagnosis was not good. I had seen my dad deal with MG and the effects of the medicine he had to take, and I would be on the same medicines: prednisone and pyridostigmine.

Within two or three weeks, my symptoms were gone completely. I remained on this dosage for about four months and began a tapering-off process designed by my MG doctor. The tapering started at 80 mg for two weeks, then 70 mg for two weeks, then 60 mg, etc., until I reached a minimum dosage of 12.5 mg of prednisone every other day and pyridostigmine only as needed. I remained on the 12.5 mg for almost two years with my MG in remission.

In September 2017, I suffered a brain aneurysm. I had to have emergency brain surgery to repair the aneurysm, and a stent was placed. Due to the trauma to my system caused by the aneurysm, my MG symptoms came back just like before. My MG doctor put me on the same medicines as before, and I started over again with prednisone (80 mg daily) and pyridostigmine, as needed. Again, the symptoms went away within a month, and I tapered off the medicines as per the doctor's plan—down to a maintenance level of 12.5 mg every other day.

In October 2018, I became ill with a bad chest cold that turned into pneumonia. My primary-care doctor put me on antibiotics to treat the cold and pneumonia. I allowed the sickness and stress to get to me. About a month into my sickness, my MG came back for the third time. This time, two new symptoms appeared: weakness in my jaw muscles and difficulty swallowing when I ate. My MG doctor upped my medicines as before: prednisone (80 mg daily) and pyridostigmine (60 mg as needed). This time, he added azathioprine (two tablets twice a day). Again, the symptoms went away, and I tapered off as per my MG doctor's plan. This time, my minimum dosage was 20 mg of prednisone every other day.

Each time I would have a relapse or episode, I would call my doctor's office, and he would see me immediately. During the treatments, I would see him once a month. During one of my visits, my wife told him how depressed I was with my recent sickness and my MG going in and out of remission. After hearing this, he put me on a mild antidepressant that has certainly helped me. I still take it every day now.

While under my MG doctor's care, I have followed the dose of the medications as directed. However, the side effects of the medications were trying for me—mainly due to the amount of medications I take for both my heart and my MG.

In summary, this is the advice from me:

- Trust your doctors; they are the experts.
- Follow your medication plan as it was designed.
- Communicate any changes that might occur to your doctor immediately.
- Manage your level of stress and depression. Don't see this as a weakness.
- Use your spouse/family to help monitor your symptoms. Likely you will know first when something changes.

Myasthenia gravis has certainly affected my quality of life, but I accept that and deal with it in my own way. I am not as strong physically as I was before and somewhat slower in my step. I try to walk each day at least two to three miles to remain active and get exercise. I believe remaining active is essential with MG; with the medications we are forced to take, being idle is another negative factor we have to deal with.

I set a goal of two to three miles, and I achieve that almost every day. I use the STEPZ application on my phone to keep track of the number of steps and the distance I walk each day. At times, I do get leg fatigue and weakness in my arms, but I try to work through it by pacing myself and taking breaks from what I am doing.

I hope my experience will help you deal with your myasthenia gravis. I accept this disease into my life now and certainly will not give in to it and let it ruin my life. I trust my doctor to get me through it, and I am grateful for his work and experience with MG.

> *"Manage your stress levels and depression, don't see this as a weakness."*

**Expert Comment:**

There are several points that are brought up by this story. When slurring of speech is the presenting symptom and develops quickly, stroke is a commonly given diagnosis. Patients may report to the ER for speech disturbances with swallowing difficulty. Brain MRI may show some age-related changes that are interpreted as consistent with stroke. Even a negative MRI of the brain does not rule out stroke. Patients receive stroke management, but symptoms continue to fluctuate and other symptoms may appear, like droopy eyelids, making the diagnosis easier.

Family history of MG is not uncommon. Family members are four times more likely to get MG than others. The disease is not hereditary, but the predisposition to it is. This may be related to the way the immune system handles challenges like infections, which are thought to be the trigger of the disease. The disease is associated with certain components of the immune system called HLA.

The disease can be exacerbated by psychological stress as well as physical stress, such as surgery, infection, heart attack, pregnancy, and delivery. During periods of stress, the maintenance dose of prednisone may need to be tripled (stressed dose). We advise patients to let their treating physician know if they are admitted to a hospital so that their dose of prednisone can be increased.

Patients who take steroids for a long time develop suppression of the adrenal glands, which produce large amounts of steroids during stress. Therefore, the body will need to receive the needed dose externally. One reason that we prescribe every other day is to avoid adrenal suppression. The adrenal glands will kick in during the steroid's off days, and that way they will not shrink.

Depression is a common complication of long-term steroid therapy, and this may present with lack of interest and disturbance of sleep and appetite. Antidepressants are helpful and do not exacerbate MG. Depressed patients tend to have poor compliance with medications and health care in general.

Mild, not fatiguing, exercises are recommended for MG patients. Immobility may increase depression and reduce muscle power. Too much activity is tiring. A balance is to be reached by each individual.

> *"Depression is a common complication of long-term steroid therapy... Antidepressants are helpful and do not exacerbate MG."*

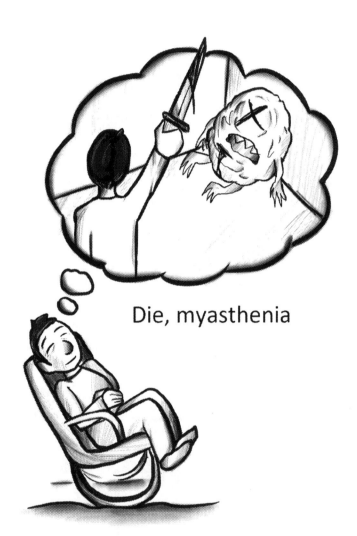

Die, myasthenia

# Case #4

## Do Not Despair, and Take Naps

"To help my psychological health, I would try to stay positive and look at what I could accomplish."

I am seventy-two years of age and was diagnosed about a year and a half ago with myasthenia gravis. My earliest symptom was that my right eye kept closing and kept feeling tired and weak. I saw my regular primary-care physician (PCP), and he wanted me to see my eye doctor. He did not believe it was Bell's palsy. I saw my eye doctor, and she suspected MG or Parkinson's disease. I asked to see an eye specialist that a friend of mine recommended, who ran tests and confirmed it was MG.

My PCP recommended a neurologist who then sent me to a trusted specialist in the disease, since MG is not common. I was concerned about the diagnosis and the consequences associated with the disease progression—one of the worst scenarios being problems with breathing and swallowing, which can be deadly.

My MG specialist was so kind and helpful when I went to my first visit. He took his time informing me about the disease and explaining how the treatment plan would go. I was given two prescriptions: one was for prednisone and the second was for Mestinon. Unfortunately, the second medication, Mestinon, gave me severe diarrhea, and so I was taken off of it. I continued with the prednisone at 80 mg per day and was given a calendar that guided my gradual decrease in the dose for the following weeks and months.

It took me about two weeks to really start feeling the effects of the medication. My right eye opened up. I could see again without blurry vision and did not have to wear an eye patch all the time. I could drive again at night, which I previously could not do anymore because of the symptoms I had. The medication also gave me energy. I felt active and exhilarated. I was not sleepy and didn't have low energy anymore.

I managed to get a lot done around my house. I am normally not an early riser, but I noticed I was up earlier in the morning after five or six hours of sleep. I had just moved into a new townhouse, and I was getting it organized. It was great! I really took advantage of feeling so good.

I have issues with my left knee and needed a complete knee replacement. My doctor had told me that the prednisone I was taking would also help my knee to feel better. My doctor was correct; I had noticed that the medication gave me relief from the pain in my knee and that I was not limping anymore. When the prednisone was dropped to 20–30 mg per day, I started to lose the high-energy level, and some pain was coming back in the left knee. I understood that prednisone can cause bad side effects over a long period of time. I wished there was a medication that worked the same way and did not have those side effects, but alas, there is not.

I was also concerned about weight gain and getting the typical moon face that people get with large doses of prednisone. I started the keto diet in January of 2019. I am also a type 2 diabetic, diagnosed three years ago. I currently take Victoza and glipizide for my type 2 diabetes. After going on the keto diet, I have lost about twenty pounds. I really do not call it a diet but more of a lifetime plan. I have not gotten the moon face, either.

> *"I was concerned…with the disease progression—one of the worst scenarios being problems with breathing and swallowing, which can be deadly."*

I thank God that my blood sugar and A1C levels are good, which I think is wonderful for someone who is on so much prednisone. I sometimes get hungry and feel like I want to eat the wallpaper off the wall, ha ha. However, I have learned how to eat the keto way with 70 percent good fats, 15 percent protein, and 15 percent carbohydrates. I have an excellent group of friends that also eat the keto way. We have developed a plan that works for us. I have lost inches and come down two clothing sizes.

I see a heart specialist in Houston, and he has done all my testing and said I am doing very well regarding my heart health. He told me to keep doing what I am doing.

I fell in early May and badly injured my right knee, which was my good knee. I now need to have surgery on it. A doctor was going to do the surgery on my knee; it was scheduled for June 12. However, I had a setback, and my right eye started to close up again four days before the surgery. I contacted my doctor who specializes in MG, and he wanted to see me. I went in a few days before I was supposed to have the surgery, and he suggested I postpone the surgery if it was not an emergency.

Needless to say, I did not want to do that. After all, I was geared up mentally for the surgery. However, after talking to my doctor more, I knew that I had to postpone. He was concerned that I would risk the possibility of having trouble during surgery with breathing or swallowing, and until I got my MG under control, we could not do the surgery. He said this could take six to eight weeks and placed me back on the 80 mg per day while also putting me on a medication called Imuran that I take three times per day to keep the symptoms under control.

I followed my doctor's orders carefully, and I did what he asked me to do. I am very grateful for my doctor, and I trust him regarding my care. As well as reading a lot on my illness, I also have a background in nursing, which allows me to understand the side effects of steroids. When I got tired, like when I was on 20 mg of prednisone a day, I just took my time doing things. I would make a list and do what I could on my list, since I could only do so much. When I got tired, I would nap or just rest. To help my psychological health, I would try to stay positive and look at what I could accomplish.

I have been taking 50 mg per day of an antidepressant known as Pristiq for years, since I have a propensity toward depression. I also see a good psychiatrist once a year for maintenance.

I have a wonderful network of friends who provide good

psychological support, and we help each other. I believe that has helped me tremendously to cope with this disease. Everything works together, I believe, for the better. God created it that way. Don't despair; we will make it with this disease. We will all help each other. That is what it is all about. Love to all of you.

> *"When the prednisone was dropped down,*
> *I started to lose the high-energy level,*
> *and some pain was coming back…"*

**Expert Comment:**

This story raises several important points. First, pyridostigmine (Mestinon) is not tolerated by some patients. It is important to know that this medicine is not supposed to change the natural course of the disease but to alleviate symptoms only for four hours after each dose. It increases the level of acetylcholine in the nerve terminal temporarily. It works in 50 percent of cases and is used for mild ocular disease or as a supplement to steroids.

If it works, it would delay the need for steroids. But even when it does work, it usually stops working after a year or two. Many patients, especially the elderly, develop intolerable side effects like muscle cramps, diarrhea, twitching of the facial muscles, and excessive salivation. Mild diarrhea usually responds to Lomotil or over the counter Imodium—one tablet an hour before the Mestinon tablet. The maximum daily dose is 540 mg.

Some patients like long-acting pyridostigmine (time span). Each tablet contains 180 mg of the active ingredient and works for twenty-four hours. I do not encourage the use of this formula because the short-acting version enables the patient to titrate the dose, and so if side effects happen, they would last only four hours.

Prednisone is the mainstay of treatment. There is no universally accepted regimen to start or to taper. I use 60–80 mg a day for six weeks followed by a tapering over three months to 10–20 mg every other day to avoid suppression of the adrenal gland. Success rate is 90 percent. Patients are usually very alarmed by what they read about side effects. Discussion about the importance of steroids and how to reduce and cope with side effects is important.

> *"Patients should know that about 10 percent of cases may worsen in the first two weeks before they get better."*

Elderly patients and those with diabetes and hypertension are at a greater risk of complications. Patients should know that about 10 percent of cases may worsen in the first two weeks before they get better. If patients have poor swallowing, speech, or breathing, the steroids may trigger respiratory failure. Therefore, if they do not live close to a medical center or are not reliable on detecting and reporting, I recommend treating them with IVIG two weeks before starting the steroids. The IVIG works within a few days and last several weeks, providing a good cover for countering initial steroid-induced worsening.

Steroids may take two to four weeks to start working. Initial side effects may include high blood pressure and blood sugar. Patients are instructed to check their BS and BP daily, especially if they are diabetics. If these are elevated, they are advised to check with their PCP to adjust their medications. Some patients need insulin during steroid therapy. Once the steroid dose is tapered, the dose of insulin is to be lowered and may well be eliminated.

Steroids may swell the lens of the eye and cause blurred vision. They may cause muscle weakness and fatigue. These symptoms are often confused by patients as MG symptoms. Patients are informed that blurred vision, muscle weakness, and fatigue will likely resolve after steroids are tapered. Yes, MG can cause these symptoms as well, but more reliable symptoms to be monitored are double vision; droopy eyelids; difficulties with swallowing, speech, and chewing; and shortness of breath.

Stomach discomfort from erosion and ulceration is more common in patients with a history of peptic ulcer. Therefore, these patients need an antacid with the steroids, like over-the-counter Pepcid, 20 mg a day. I use vitamin D 1,000 IU a day and calcium gluconate 1,000 mg a day with steroids to reduce the risk of osteoporosis, and I check bone density every year in females and every two years in males. If osteoporosis develops, I would refer them for treatment to an internist.

After the steroid is initiated, I ask for a follow-up in three weeks to monitor side effects, then after another three weeks to start tapering. Long-term side effects include osteoporosis, cataract, and skin striation. Increased appetite and weight gain are common. Weight gain can be caused by fluid retention as well, and that may be treated with diuretics. Since both steroids and diuretics can cause loss of potassium, I encourage my patients to eat two bananas a day and to check their serum potassium periodically.

Insomnia, anxiety, depression, and palpitation are other common side effects. Redistribution of body fat may lead to buffalo hump (accumulation of fat behind the neck) and moon face. Patients follow different dietary regimens, but the key is to reduce carbohydrate intake and to mildly exercise.

The issue of exercise in MG is tricky. MG and steroids cause fatigue. We encourage patients to do mild exercises like walking and swimming and to avoid excessive exposure to heat.

Elective surgery is not recommended until MG is under control with minimum medications. Poorly controlled MG may be exacerbated by surgery and prolonged intubation, leading to more complications. High-dose steroids may delay healing and increase the risk of infection.

> *"Elective surgery is not recommended until MG is under control with minimum medications."*

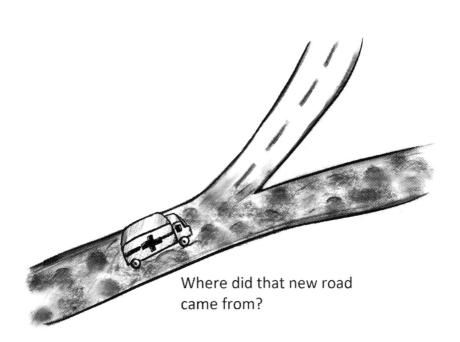

Where did that new road came from?

# Case #5

## A Miracle Happened

I am seventy-six years old. I was diagnosed with myasthenia gravis on March 2, 2018. Prior to this date, my only serious health problems were wet macular degeneration in the right eye, diagnosed in 2005, and prostate cancer, diagnosed in 2009. I later had the prostate removed.

My symptoms of MG started around Thanksgiving 2017. The first symptom that I noticed was that while lying in bed at night, I tried to swallow and could not. I would have to try around ten times, and then finally I could swallow. This went on for several nights.

A couple of weeks went by, and I noticed that I was starting to have problems with food going down my throat. It seemed like the opening of my throat was smaller. The food would go down, but I could tell that there was something different about my throat opening.

One day, right after eating, I went out to the driveway. I bent over to pick something up, and all my food from lunch came up. It did not look like vomit; it was as if the food I just ate for lunch came out like I ate it. That started to get me concerned.

I then started thinking about going to my gastrologist to get my upper GI system checked to see what was wrong. All the procedures and tests to check my GI system took about a month. During that time, my speech was starting to slur, and my tongue felt different with the slurring of the speech. I was starting to think I'd had a stroke or something to do with the brain.

I made an appointment with my cardiologists. Both the cardiologist and gastrologist found nothing wrong. The gastrologist made me an appointment with a neurologist. It took about a month to get the appointment. During this time, I continued to have the same symptoms and some additional weakness in my arms. I was checked out by the cardiologist, and he said everything was okay. There was no indication of a stroke, and there were no other concerns.

By this time, we were getting into February, and my arms and legs were starting to feel weak. My right eye was also starting to droop. I was very concerned and frustrated, because no doctor could tell me what my problem was. I had a couple of bad falls, and that was really concerning to me.

So, we are now up to March 2, when I went to see a neurologist. He interviewed me for about ten minutes, and then he told me that I have MG. He then made an appointment for me one week later, March 12, 2018, with a specialist in a bigger city.

The day after I left the neurologist, I was in the driveway, walking to go pick up the mail, when I suddenly collapsed. My wife could not pick me up, so I asked her to call 911. We felt like we needed to find something out soon, because in a day or two, I would not be able to walk. I chose to go to a specific hospital because the MG specialist was there.

Once 911 was called, the two attendants came to get me and take me to a hospital in the city. When I was on the way to a particular hospital, one of the EMTs received a call from that hospital saying that I was being rerouted to a different hospital because they were full. I didn't know it at the time, but this was one of the biggest miracles that happened to me during my fight with MG.

At about 7 p.m., I made it to the hospital and went straight to my assigned room. Around 9 p.m., I was awakened by a doctor and four interns. This doctor was teaching a class on MG, and I was going to be used as a patient for MG training. This is why I referred to the rerouting to a different hospital as a miracle. I was told by the doctor that I had all the classic symptoms of the disease. I was also told that the blood pressure medication I had been taking for over thirty years, atenolol, was on the list of medications to avoid for MG.

I was then asked if I was up to having tests done all night so they could rule out other causes of MG. They asked me to be ready in the morning so they could start feeding me a solution that would help me get back on my feet. Some of the blood was used to make this feeding solution. I told him I would do whatever needed to be done. He said he had to rule out other things that could be causing the disease and that it would probably take all night.

He was right. By the time they got through with me in the morning, I was really exhausted. At that point, I had done a total of two hours and twenty minutes inside the MRI machine.

The next morning, the doctor came into my room to tell me that the results were good and that they were going to start feeding me the solution they'd made using a feeding tube through my nose and into my stomach. I lived on that solution for five days. After five days, the doctor removed the feeding tube, and I spent a day walking around trying to get my strength back. Finally, on Friday, I was released to go home. I was told to stay on 60 mg of prednisone per day until my next appointment, which would be two weeks from that Friday with a different MG specialist.

When I saw my new MG specialist for the first time, he gave me a chart showing the amount of prednisone to take each day; he was trying to slowly wean me off it. Once I was down to 15 mg, though, my symptoms started to come back. The doctor told me that I would have to start over at 60 mg of prednisone in addition to 20 mg of methotrexate, to be taken once a week on the same day of each week. Currently, I am down to 20 mg of prednisone, which I take every other day, and 20 mg of methotrexate, which I take one day a week.

During the time when I was coming off of the prednisone, most of my symptoms slowly went away. The only symptom that persists is my eyes. My vision is not what it was prior to MG. I was diagnosed by a retinal specialist with wet macular degeneration in both eyes. I don't know if this can be attributed to MG.

So as of today, June 13, I am on 20 mg of prednisone every other day and 20 mg of methotrexate taken one day a week on the same day each week. I have been on this dosage for several weeks with no symptoms of MG.

> *"I was told that the blood pressure medication I had been taking for over thirty years, atenolol, was on the list of medications to avoid for MG."*

**Expert Comment:**

Symptoms of MG can mimic several disorders and can progress dramatically. When swallowing difficulty is the only feature, patients undergo a full workup to rule out gastrointestinal problems. When slurring of speech is the main issue, then a stroke workup is initiated. If shortness of breath is the presenting symptom, the respiratory and cardiac systems are the focus of investigation. Droopy eyelids and fatigability of chewing are fairly characteristic of MG and should prompt the right workup immediately. Fatigability of chewing is painless, unlike painful chewing due to TMJ pain. If the pain is in the jaw muscles, a condition called *temporal arteritis* has to be kept in mind. This condition can cause blindness and stroke and is treatable. It is not directly related to MG.

When symptoms recur during steroid tapering, a steroid-sparing agent is added. In this case, methotrexate was chosen. This medication is used to treat some cancers and autoimmune diseases like rheumatoid arthritis. It blocks the formation of folic acid, which is necessary for the formation of new inflammatory cells. It has many other anti-inflammatory properties. It may take a month or two to start working. Folic acid 1 mg a day is recommended to prevent folic acid deficiency. Its dosing is convenient as a once-weekly oral or subcutaneous injection.

Rarely, patients may develop fibrosis of the lungs with subsequent shortness of breath that can be confused as caused by MG. A CAT scan of the chest should resolve the confusion. After two years, the dose is to be gradually reduced to see if a lasting remission has been achieved. Most patients with MG will require some kind of maintenance therapy for years.

Blurred vision in a patient with MG does not have to be caused by MG. Cataract, glaucoma, macular degeneration, and increased intracranial pressure should all be considered. An ophthalmology consult would be appropriate.

> **"When symptoms recur during steroid tapering, a steroid-sparing agent is added. In this case, methotrexate was chosen... which has many anti-inflammatory properties."**

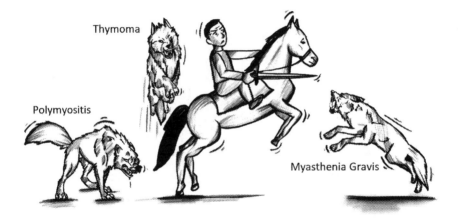
Polymyositis

Thymoma

Myasthenia Gravis

# Case #6

## FINDINGS DID NOT MAKE SENSE TO MY DOCTOR

It was the middle of June 1999. I woke up with a headache, which was unusual, because I didn't normally get headaches. I didn't have a fever, but my muscles felt sore, and I had very little energy. I figured if I rested a few days, I would regain my stamina. That didn't happen. Each day, I felt worse.

After about a week, my wife drove me to our family doctor. He immediately had me admitted to a hospital. I had been there two days when it was concluded that I had experienced a stroke. My wife and I politely disagreed. Okay, we weren't very polite.

After that brouhaha, a doctor who was not directly involved in diagnosing my case said that he would refer me to a neurologist. We readily agreed.

At the hospital, the neurologist came to examine me. I told him how my weakness and exhaustion had come upon me suddenly. I showed him that I could not stand on my tiptoes. He listened to my nasal Donald Duck (my wife's term) voice, and then he poured me some cold water and had me slowly sip it. My voice came back to normal.

He said that he was pretty sure that I had myasthenia gravis, but that he wanted to run some confirmation tests. He checked me out of the hospital because he knew no tests would be done over the Fourth of July weekend.

After a long weekend of worrying and conjecture, the tests began. They indicated myasthenia gravis. A scan showed that I had an enlarged thymus gland. It had to go. My neurologist gave me a muscle biopsy, which indicated that I also had polymyositis. He prescribed Mestinon to be taken before meals so that I could chew and swallow. He also prescribed a high dosage of prednisone to build up my strength for a thymectomy.

On September 17, 1999, I was lying on a gurney at the hospital waiting to enter the operating room. One of the anesthesiologists asked me how I was doing. I said, "I'd rather be fishing, and I don't even like to fish!" I don't remember anything between there and waking up in the recovery room. Thanks to the surgeon and many others, the operation was a success. In fact, it was so successful that the doctors at a radiation clinic decided I didn't need radiation therapy.

After the operation, I received IVIG treatments along with prednisone, Imuran (azathioprine), and other medicine. In a few months, I was actually able to get on my tractor and drive it. In fact, through my neurologist's association with the local news station, I was shown on TV driving the tractor!

I now take only the minimum doses of medicine that my neurologist thinks I need. I feel pretty good, have good strength, and can do most of the things that I used to do. My wife and I owe a great debt of thanks to my doctor and all his staff. We shall forever be grateful.

> *"After the thymectomy, I received IVIG treatments along with...other medicine. In a few months, I was able to drive my tractor."*

**Expert Comment:**

This patient had a very unusual combination of myasthenia gravis, polymyositis (muscle inflammation), and thymoma (tumor of the thymus gland). His arm and leg weakness was more than what could be expected for MG, and his muscle enzyme (CK) was very high, suggesting muscle inflammation, which was confirmed by a muscle biopsy that also showed some strange cells called *giant cells* because they are very big and have many nuclei. That is why it is called *giant cell myositis.*

Fortunately, his thymoma was not malignant and was taken care of by removal of the thymus. Treatment of MG and polymyositis was undertaken with the same agents (prednisone and azathioprine), and severe symptoms were treated with IVIG. The patient led almost a normal life except for an exacerbation of symptoms when azathioprine was discontinued three years later. He had severe slurring of speech and chewing fatigability. He had to hold his lower jaw with his right hand to be able to chew effectively. He had droopy eyelids and double vision and some dysphagia. Symptoms were then controlled by reintroduction of the azathioprine and increasing prednisone to 80 mg a day.

All the reported cases (only a few) in the literature were grim due to involvement of the heart with this inflammatory process (carditis). Fortunately, he did not have carditis. Every now and then, he used pyridostigmine for swallowing and chewing difficulty. He managed his disease well. His wife, who was his caregiver, had cancer of the pancreas. She died within six months. Within a month, he had a headache and was found to have an aggressive brain tumor called *glioblastoma*. He died six months later. Azathioprine increases the risk of cancer if used for a long time. That is why every two to three years, weaning is tried. Stress may unmask cancer.

> **"Azathioprine may increase the risk of cancer if used for a long time."**

Double vision. No problem,
its double food

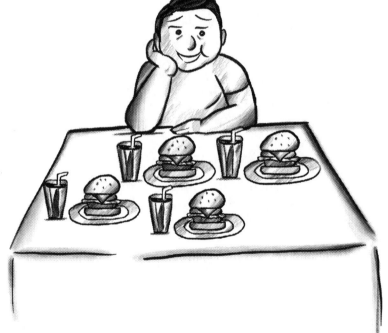

# Case #7

## DELAYED DIAGNOSIS

"Due to the vague and transient nature of the symptoms of MG…
It is not unusual for it to take a year for the diagnosis to be made."

Some of my earliest symptoms included slight trouble with the ability to focus my vision. However, rapid eye blinking seemed to restore my normal vision. Later on, this did not help much, and better eyesight was obtained by squinting one or both eyelids. When the double vision started, I tried to cancel it by mentally concentrating like people would when reading without their glasses. This worked to correct the double vision, but I could not keep it up. Once I relaxed, the double vision would return. My double vision worsened along with a worsening of my sense of depth perception. My left eye was most affected and began to turn to the left.

> *"Due to the vague and transient nature of the symptoms of MG…It is not unusual for it to take a year for the diagnosis to be made."*

Another thing I did to obtain higher-quality eyesight more quickly was to close the left eye when needed. When the right eye was closed and the left eye was open, a loss of balance occurred, so care was used to prevent falling or injury. Going from bright to dark areas took longer to adjust to. Partially covering the left eye with a patch would almost get rid of double vision, and I would use this to help me most of the time. Also, you can train yourself to use your best eye even when both eyes are uncovered. You can do this by training yourself to ignore the vision coming from the worst eye. Another symptom I noticed was some loss of body strength.

Some ways I coped with the symptoms was moving slower and using extra caution when driving by using the partial eye patch on the most affected eye. Not only did my hand–eye coordination suffer but so did my reading, making tasks more difficult.

It took about eight months, several doctors, and many tests before a diagnosis was made. My symptoms started to slowly go away, even with the minimum amount of Mestinon that I was taking just when needed. I had no problems for over a year, but then gradually symptoms began to return.

When hearing the diagnosis, I reacted okay, but I was concerned about the possibility of a major surgery. This worry was short-term, since I had good test results and the medication proved to be successful because my symptoms went into remission. The first treatment was Mestinon, and since I had the minimum dosage of the medication, I had no side effects. However, when the maximum dosage was later used, my body muscles started twitching, and I experienced a lack of energy and diarrhea. This medication helped but did not correct the double vision.

The second treatment I started taking was prednisone. There was no change until around the tenth day. From there, I would have good and bad days, but after two weeks, I began to see good results. After three weeks, my vision was normal, but I did experience some side effects, which are mentioned below:

- constipation, but not excessive
- increase in appetite
- weight gain
- slight upset stomach and bitter taste in my mouth
- tremors in arms and hands starting around six hours after taking morning medication
- shortness of breath during mild exercise
- loss of taste

> ## *"Partially covering the left eye with a patch would almost get rid of double vision."*

**Expert Comment:**

Double vision is a common presentation of MG. It occurs to one or more directions of gaze and is typically more severe during visual activity like reading and watching TV and in the evening. It gets better with rest. There is no associated numbness or tingling of the face or severe headache. These symptoms would suggest a brain process such as blood clot or tumor. Characteristically, the double vision disappears when either eye is closed.

Patients learn many tricks to avoid double vision. During driving, an upcoming strong light may trigger double vision because the eye muscles cannot accommodate effectively. This may cause car accidents. Patients are advised to have an eye patch in the car all the time.

Due to the vague and transient nature of the symptoms of MG, diagnosis is delayed. It is not unusual for it to take a year for the diagnosis to be made. Symptoms may go away on their own in 20 percent of cases. Pyridostigmine helps the double vision for four hours, and the dose can be increased to a maximum of 120 mg (two tablets) every four to six hours when needed. It is not a bad idea to take pyridostigmine an hour before driving if double vision is an issue. Side effects—including diarrhea, muscle cramps, and muscle twitching—may limit pyridostigmine use.

Prednisone is the mainstay of treatment for MG. Side effects are common but usually mild and tolerated, and they almost always resolve when the dose is decreased. All the mentioned symptoms are real. Body weight, blood pressure, blood sugar, bone density, and vision should be monitored during steroid therapy.

Cataract is a common long-term side effect. Blurring of vision is not always a sign of relapse of myasthenia. Steroids may swell the lens and cause the blurring. Cataract, glaucoma and increased intracranial pressure are other possibilities caused by or worsened by steroids. Therefore, when blurring of vision occurs, especially with headache and with no double vision or swallowing or speech difficulty, an eye examination by an ophthalmologist and a brain MRI would be appropriate.

Likewise, increasing shortness of breath is not always a feature of MG exacerbation. Heart failure triggered by uncontrolled high blood pressure due to steroid therapy, fluid retention worsened by steroids, weight gain, and exacerbation of pulmonary tuberculosis by steroids should be considered when shortness of breath is not associated with double vision or swallowing difficulty.

> **"Prednisone is the mainstay
> of treatment for MG."**

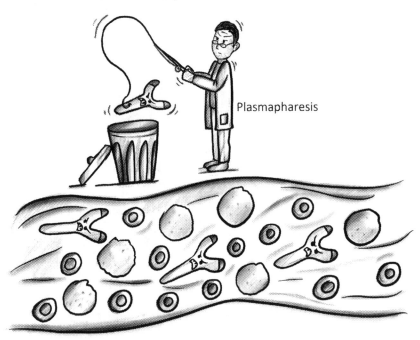

# Case #8

## NOTHING SEEMS TO WORK

"Patients who do not respond to or tolerate steroids or
chemotherapy may need to be on PLEX or IVIG for years."

In early 2007, I noticed my left eyelid was drooping, and it was very
tired and weak. As time went on, my eyelid was mostly closed, and I was
getting too weak to work. After seeing the company doctor, I was sent to
an ophthalmologist who examined my eyes and asked me some questions
about my health problems. By this time, I was so weak, and I was having
trouble breathing, chewing, and swallowing. I was sent for an acetylcholine
blood test, as one doctor suspected I had myasthenia gravis. A few days
later, I was told the number from the test was so high that it would kill
me unless I got treatment.

I was sent to a neurologist, who quickly prescribed Mestinon and
prednisone. After being on these medications, I wasn't improving; in fact,
I was getting worse. The neurologist then started me on IVIG treatment
along with the same meds. I didn't improve much over the next year and
was given different medications that either caused other problems or didn't
work. Finally, along with the IVIG treatment, I was put on some chemo
pills. I was starting to feel a little stronger and was slightly improving. After
a few months, I was taken off the IVIG treatment but continued with the
two prescriptions. About six months later, I started urinating blood, since

the chemo pills were damaging my bladder. I was taken off the chemo and was now only on Mestinon.

It's now mid–2010, and my health goes straight downhill over a few days. I am so weak that I can't even talk. Of course, breathing, chewing, swallowing, and double vision are all a major problem now. I was given five consecutive days of IVIG treatment and another acetylcholine blood test. The test numbers were even higher than they were in 2007. I was then sent to an MG specialist for plasmapheresis treatment and evaluation.

I am still on plasmapheresis today along with taking Mestinon. Since being treated by my MG doctor, I have had a thymectomy, tried different medications, and even had an experimental infusion. In September 2011, I had a relapse and was on life support for seven days and in the hospital for eleven days. I received six consecutive days of plasmapheresis while on life support.

As of 2019, I am still affected by myasthenia gravis. I have trouble chewing at times and still need a lot of rest. Breathing isn't very good, especially when I walk more than normal. I'm not very active anymore and have learned what my limit is. I'm very thankful for the care that my MG doctor has given me through the years. At least I'm maintaining and can function to a certain degree with the plasmapheresis treatment.

> *"...I started urinating blood, since the chemo pills were damaging my bladder."*

**Expert Comment:**

While it is true that the disease can kill if neglected, the level of acetylcholine receptor antibody titer does not correlate with the severity of the disease. It is used for diagnosis and not for follow-up of the disease activity. Less than 7 percent of cases are refractory. They just do not respond or tolerate pyridostigmine, steroids, IVIG, and chemotherapy (azathioprine, cyclosporine, methotrexate, mycophenolate, cyclophosphamide, etc.).

Plasma exchange (PLEX) has been proven to be effective. The blood is taken from a vein and fed into a machine that will eliminate the plasma, replace it with normal saline, and reinfuse it through an artery. The procedure is usually done in the hospital on an outpatient basis. PLEX is as effective as IVIG, which can be done in any infusion center or even a patient's home. However, PLEX works faster, and it may succeed when IVIG fails. Both are temporizing agents and are given in severe cases until steroids and chemotherapy start working (weeks to months, respectively).

Patients who do not respond to or tolerate steroids or chemotherapy may need to be on PLEX or IVIG for years. This may mandate an AV shunt, similar to the one used for dialysis or a PIC line, to avoid puncturing a peripheral vein every visit. With time, peripheral veins become fragile and inaccessible. Some patients need PLEX every week, others every one to three months. PLEX may cause low blood pressure or low serum calcium, or disturb heart rhythm during the procedure. However, with good intravenous hydration, addition of calcium, and proper positioning of the central cath, these complications can be minimized. The central line or the AV shunt may get obstructed periodically. However, this problem is manageable.

> **"Less than 7 percent of cases are refractory."**

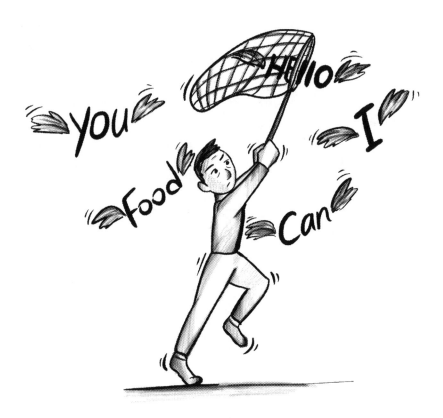

I am losing my speech!

# Case #9

## THANK YOU, JESUS

"If I have any changes in medication, I
keep my neurologist informed."

In January of 2008, I was experiencing what I thought was tiredness in my eyes. I would rub my eyes vigorously because it seemed to make them feel better.

In August of 2008, I woke up on a Sunday morning with a definite slur in my speech. Thinking I might be having a stroke, I checked my extremities and found I had all my functions. I took a shower, shaved, and brushed my teeth. When I tried to spit out the toothpaste, I realized I couldn't spit. I tried to wash out my mouth and found I couldn't slosh the water in my mouth. When I leaned over the sink to spit the water out, the water just fell out of my mouth.

Several hours later, a family friend who is a doctor instructed me to go to the emergency room at a local hospital. The ER staff was waiting for me when I arrived and quickly ushered me into a room. From Sunday afternoon until the following Tuesday, they ran every test imaginable, minus a pregnancy test.

The specialist assigned to my case came in my room and informed me that he had no idea what was going on. He wanted me to go to the city to consult with a neurologist. On Wednesday morning, I went to the center, where I saw and met with the neurologist. After discussing with the doctor my experiences over the past four days, I was asked to come back in two weeks.

I returned home on Thursday morning and returned to work on regular duty (my speech was the only thing impaired). Within the next six days, I began to experience difficulty breathing and swallowing, and what I thought was weakness in my neck, arms, and legs. In the first episode with swallowing difficulties, I lost thirty-nine pounds in seven days because I refused a feeding tube. I was getting fluids intravenously during those seven days. I contacted the neurologist's office at the request of my plant nurse, and they scheduled me the next morning.

After listening to my concerns, my neurologist scheduled a blood test and two other tests (I don't recall what they were called). At the completion of the final test, I was diagnosed with myasthenia gravis. My diagnosis took approximately two weeks.

My reaction to the diagnosis was concern, but I really liked my neurologist and trusted him completely. I concluded, from his information, that this was a process that was going to take some time, but with his help, I would get through this and live a normal life. In terms of my psychological state, I admit there were days when I had a pity party. It's not fun having this disease, but I never wanted to be treated like I was sick. On bad days, I allowed my wife to help me, but I never stopped helping myself (it helps to be a positive person). I could always find someone worse off than I was.

Even with the symptoms I was experiencing, I was able to continue with my job and all my day-to-day activities. I seemed to tire easily but continued to function pretty close to normal. Having consulted with my neurologist, I was assured that the myasthenia gravis was treatable, and I could live a normal life.

The first treatment was a high dose of a steroid called prednisone. I informed my neurologist that in no way would I ever consent to taking a steroid. What I had heard about steroids was not favorable (my lack of knowledge). After much discussion and my continued refusal to take the steroid, I returned home and continued to work and live with my symptoms. My doctor did inform me that eventually I would take the steroid, but he allowed me to leave without the prescription.

I lost thirty-nine pounds in seven days, I was struggling enormously, trying to work and carry on life as before. I finally consented to take the steroid, reluctantly. I was informed that I would probably crash before I got better. I did.

The following day, I took the steroid, prednisone (80 mg), and within an hour, I lost the ability to swallow. I couldn't even swallow my own saliva. About five hours after taking the prednisone (while at work), I tried to take a drink of water. I aspirated on it, couldn't get my breath, became unconscious, and woke up in our medical department with an ambulance on the way to pick me up and bring me to a local hospital. My neurologist was notified and ordered an IVIG.

I was in the ICU for six days and received a total of five bags in five days. I believe it helped me tremendously, and I don't recall any bad side effects from the IVIG. I was told I might have headaches, but I didn't. I don't recall having any other treatments, but if I did, they undoubtedly did some good. After I recovered from my first episode with swallowing difficulties, I don't recall any recurrences of that issue. My neurologist is a caring doctor, and without his guidance, I wouldn't be where I am today: fully recovered.

I eventually did suffer a relapse one year and one month from my original diagnosis. I then had a thymectomy and experienced a third relapse three years later. The cause was reducing my dosage of prednisone too much too soon. I was in agreement with the aggressive dosage reduction. I understood that we tried, but it didn't work. I didn't like the results, but I stayed in the battle and continued to fight.

My thymectomy was a little more complicated than most because the thymus had connected itself to other organs and tissue. The surgeon was successful in getting it all. I experienced no bad side effects with the thymectomy.

When it came to my medication dosing, I trusted my doctor completely and never deviated from the instructions given as to the amount and the frequency. I started with 80 mg once a day, and I am currently at 2.5 mg every other day. Listen to your MG specialist; they have a plan, and I know it worked for me.

The steroids did increase my appetite, and I gained about twenty-five pounds. I have since lost the extra pounds, and I feel great. The benefit of the steroids was that they started me on the road to recovery. The side effects for me was that the prednisone increased my appetite.

If I have any changes in medication, I keep my neurologist informed. My family physician is completely engaged with my MG issues, as is my dentist, and they stay current with my progress. I do have a list of different medications and provide my neurologist with an up-to-date list of all medications and dosages. I stay in constant contact with his office and update him on any changes that take place.

My myasthenia did not affect my daily physical activity. I am as active as I ever was. I have been able to exercise as frequently as I want. When it came to the fatigue, I would take more breaks if I needed to. I've learned to not overdo it as often. I work as hard as I ever did, just not as long. I take the time to cool off more often. I just get the rest I feel I need each day.

I believe I am a positive person and always try to find the good in every situation. I've always had a strong faith in God and believe His Word concerning healing. I trust my neurologist and believe God put him in my path for such a time as this, but my hope was not in him. I thank God every day for my doctor and pray God's blessing on him. I know God was with me throughout this whole ordeal, and I'm thankful he placed my neurologist in my path. I will always be grateful.

Thank you, Jesus, and thank you to my doctor and his staff for all y'all do for so many people. You are a blessing. You are an effect of the blessing on my life.

> **"When it came to the fatigue, I would take more breaks if I needed to."**

**Expert Comment:**

This case raises the following points:

- Morning symptoms: Symptoms of MG are more severe toward the end of the day. Usually the symptoms are mild or not present early in the morning. They appear after the patient resumes activity. Sometimes they appear in the second half of the day, but in severe cases, they may appear within an hour after awakening. However, rarely, symptoms express themselves right after awakening. This is more so in patients with insomnia or poor sleep due to apnea or other factors. Nevertheless, if the symptoms appear in the morning and improve toward the end of the day, the diagnosis of MG should be questioned.

- Symptoms may progress dramatically. They may start with mild drooping of the eyelids, but soon after, they are followed by double vision, swallowing and speech difficulty, and shortness of breath. Such a dramatic progression is always an indication for an emergency evaluation and management, because respiratory failure is a real possibility and may happen quickly. We educate our patients about the importance of such a progression and more so of swallowing and speech difficulty as precursors of respiratory failure. These should never be ignored.

- Onset and progression of symptoms may be triggered by certain drugs used for treatment of other conditions, such as antibiotics like ciprofloxacin or streptomycin, seizure medications like phenytoin, or medications for disturbed heart rhythm like quinine. Sometimes an eyedrop of medications like neomycin can trigger a myasthenic crisis (respiratory failure). Patients should keep a list of offensive medications and should ask their treating physician before starting any if they have a doubt.

- Job modification: Myasthenia is a chronic disease that is treatable, but most patients will have some fatigability and lack of stamina. It all depends on the kind of job. Certainly, outdoor activities are to be limited, as MG can be triggered by heat. Jobs that require repetitive movement, such as shrimp peeling or typing, may become difficult to perform. Sedentary jobs are recommended as long as the space is air-conditioned. High-volume phone calls may be hard to handle by a myasthenic receptionist. It is important to evaluate patients in the light of their symptoms and the type of job.

---

> *"If the symptoms appear in the morning*
> *and improve toward the end of the day, the*
> *diagnosis of MG should be questioned."*

---

- Type of physical activity and exercises that patients with MG can do depend on the severity of the symptoms. We recommend against strenuous activity during steroid therapy due to fatigue and palpitation. Return to normal activity is possible after the medications are minimized, but that would depend on the definition of normal activity for that specific patient. Two to thirty minutes of walking or swimming a day is usually tolerated. If normal activity means heavy weightlifting, that may need to be adjusted.

- IVIG is very effective and is indicated for severe cases or those in myasthenic crisis. A crisis is defined by severe bulbar dysfunction (respiratory and swallowing difficulty). IVIG starts working within hours. It consists of antibodies collected from a pool of plasma collected from many people. These antibodies are supposed to attack the antibodies that the system generates against the muscle. However, their effects usually last a few weeks, and they will have to be repeated every two to six weeks depending on the case response. They are given intravenously over several hours a day for two days, followed by one day every two to six weeks. Side effects are not common except mild headache and flulike reactions. Rare but more serious side effects may include venous thrombosis, renal failure, heart attack, skin rash, and meningitis.

  IVIG can be used as a long-term therapy in patients who cannot tolerate or do not respond to steroids and chemotherapy. One important consideration for IVIG is when a patient has swallowing and chewing difficulty started on steroids. In 7 percent of cases, patients may worsen to a degree that they cannot swallow or chew, and they may develop breathing problems. These cases may be initiated with IVIG along with steroids, thus providing coverage for the possible steroid-induced worsening.

- Thymectomy has been practiced for fifty years in MG, but only it became evidence-based in 2016 when a large and long controlled trial confirmed its utility. Removal of the thymus is indicated not only in patients with tumor of the gland (thymoma) but in all patients with MG if the symptoms spread beyond the eyes. Thymectomy starts working after a year, and it will reduce the dose of prednisone and other medications needed to suppress the disease. It may reduce the risk of exacerbation and admission to the hospital and the number of patients who remain in remission without medications in the long run. Thymectomy can be done through a sternal split or through a scope introduced from the side of the chest. Complications are rare and include bleeding and poor healing.

• Importance of faith in healing depends on how one practices it. A patient of mine stopped all medications because she saw Jesus in her sleep telling her that he'd healed her. She came in a couple of weeks later with respiratory failure. Probably she brought that dream to herself by thinking that she was healed and could get away with stopping the treatment.

However, many of my patients use faith as a complementary measure along with the medical instructions. I have noticed that faith provides them with strength and purpose to endure the difficulties created by such an unpredictable disease. It alleviates their anxiety.

Faith may provides patients with strength and purpose. Second-guessing everything the doctor says and not trusting the doctor's judgment may have a negative impact on the healing process. Some patients change the dose and frequency of the medications on their own, and they only learn after the disease gets exacerbated and they have to go to the ER once or twice.

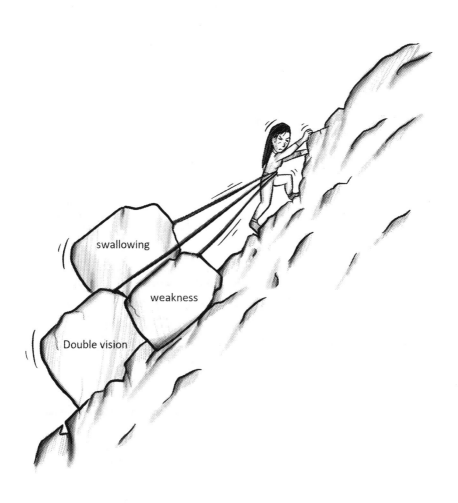

# Case #10

## So Many Symptoms

The spring of 1998 marked the downward spiral of my "perfect" health. I was forty-three years old and was working in multiple medical facilities in a large metropolitan city where MARSA, pneumonia, tuberculosis, and hepatitis B and C exposure was rampant and mandatory shots were required for employees. Shortly after receiving a series of very cold and painful hepatitis B shots, I came down with a three-week illness that I believe triggered the myasthenia gravis (ocular) symptoms.

During the next few months after those shots, I began to experience double vision and diplopia (drooping upper eyelid) in one eye. A visit to my ophthalmologist was uneventful. I was given a patch to put over my eye and told to rest for two weeks. As time passed, not only was this treatment not improving my vision, but the symptoms were exacerbating. The double vision occurred daily along with diplopia; in addition, I frequently choked on food and had painful lightning-bolt sensations shooting out of my eyes.

Although it was difficult and frustrating to work, see, and drive, this did not stop me. I kept working for three to four months, planning and hosting a bat mitzvah for my daughter and cochairing a conference for my nursing home. When these commitments were finalized, I scheduled an initial visit, in September of 1998, to see a neurologist at a hospital in my city.

After a physical exertion test was completed, blood was taken, and an edrophonium (Tensilon) test was administered, the neurologist felt that I needed immediate additional testing. Since the weekend was approaching, he sent me downstairs to the emergency room triage to have paperwork

93

filled out, interviews, more blood work, and several spinal taps on the lower part of my back. At this time, MG (ocular) was confirmed.

I was transferred upstairs to one of the clinical observation floors, where I received a battery of tests, MRIs, and visitations by medical students and doctors wanting to know more about me and my MG. No prescribed medication was given to me during this time outside of a sleeping pill. I must confess, at this time, I was scared and nervous about my future. Would I be able to continue working, or would I have to go on disability? Most importantly, who was going to care for my family, my husband, and my two children, ages thirteen and nine? I couldn't see, swallow, sleep, focus, or ambulate without getting dizzy or disoriented.

Basically, over the next three to four days, I lay in a hospital bed being prodded and awakened every two hours by someone standing over me discussing my symptoms. Thymectomy surgery was deemed not necessary at this time. My discharge procedure was brief and lacked emotional and community support. They were sending me home with the following medications: prednisone, pyridostigmine bromide, and a pill for my vertigo.

Eventually, as I was laid up at home with limited information and a lack of network community support, anger and disappointment set in due to the insensitivity and lack of support shown to me by the doctors during my treatment. Fortunately, within a week, my symptoms began to improve. The vertigo went away, my eyelids opened, and the double vision decreased.

> *"I joined an MG internet group…This network interaction gave me hope and strength to beat this disease or at least get it under control."*

Several weeks later, I consulted with the old neurologist. He took me off the pyridostigmine bromide, because the medication was causing severe diarrhea and abdominal pain, but he left me on a high dosage of steroids. Outside of the human resources department calling me for a follow-up, there was minimal communication with the hospital neurologist I saw that day, except for a few visits and the reordering of steroids. Clearly, it was time to find a new neurologist.

With my limited knowledge about this disease, and having no one to talk to or compare symptoms with, I joined an MG internet group and began chatting with hundreds of individuals who were diagnosed with a variety of symptoms. This network interaction was rewarding and informative, giving me hope and strength to beat this disease or at least get it under control. I was able to return to work within two weeks and was stabilized on the prednisone outside of the side effects of weight gain and moodiness.

Although I had been battling this serious autoimmune neuromuscular disease for a short period of time, I stayed positive and took control of my life the best I knew how. Because this disease only affected my vision (ocular MG), I still had the physical strength and endurance to stay active. Priding myself on being healthy, and to alleviate the weight gain and moodiness, I got myself back into a walking, weight training, and meditation program.

I discovered that all the data showed that long-term use of prednisone might lead to osteoporosis, thinning skin, bruising easily, and increased risk of infections. Therefore, I had a dialogue with my new neurologist, two years after being diagnosed, about reducing the steroid dosage. Over the next five years, while being monitored by the neurologist, I made attempts to cut back on the prednisone, with poor results and visual issues. Finally, after five or six years (2003), I was successful in getting off the prednisone and stayed in remission.

When I was in my mid-fifties (2008), menopause slowly kicked in, which started an avalanche of unwanted (maybe predisposed) symptoms: high blood pressure, high cholesterol, and low thyroid. Three new medications were prescribed: levothyroxine, Lisinopril, and simvastatin. Along with these new medications, as well as a colonoscopy and a flu shot, my MG symptoms reappeared. I had a serious relapse. It seemed like my autoimmune system was compromised.

This time, I anticipated the symptoms and made an appointment with a new neurologist (the old one had moved). I was put back on prednisone, on which I stayed for the next three to four years (2012) with minimal vision issues. I was having blood work monitored by my general physician every six months to monitor my lipid panels and kidney function. At times, there were problematic issues with my blood work, which showed high triglycerides, bad HDL levels, and stress with my kidneys. All of these symptoms were closely monitored over the next year. My doctor and I had a dialogue about finding another alternative medication, other than prednisone, due to the serious long-term side effects, but unfortunately, there were no other options.

During the next three to four years (2012–2014), my double vision was fluctuating along with blurriness, dry eyes, and tingling in my fingers and toes. I was increasingly getting sick and experiencing achy bone pain all over my body. Additionally, I had difficulty sleeping and was restless. I made an appointment to see a neuro-ophthalmologist at a wellness center in my city for alternative treatments to improve my vision. Many eye exams were performed, and I was told that I had severe dry eyes. Short-term treatment was a two-week regimen of prescribed eyedrops. I was given a sleeping mask with cold packets to put inside at bedtime and in the morning.

When this treatment didn't reduce the double vision and blurriness, the doctor sent me to several other eye specialists, and I even had an MRI done for my eye. Nothing corrected the double vision, and I was fitted with a prism to place over the left lens of my glasses so I could work and drive.

The neuro-ophthalmologist referred me to a new neurologist (around 2015). Although I thought this new neurologist had a fresh approach to treating my MG, it came at a time when my finances were limited, and I lost my private medical insurance when my husband went on Medicare. It became difficult to maintain ongoing six-week visits, take time off from work, and pay for medication changes (prednisone, mycophenolate, biotin). An MRI was recommended for a baseline assessment, but I couldn't afford the out-of-pocket expense.

I did manage to purchase a Health Insurance Marketplace plan, but it didn't cover specialists, which included neurologists. I was waiting out the eight months until I became eligible for Medicare. During this time, I was unable to see my general physician and neurologist, since they weren't on the "list."

Over those eight months, my symptoms exacerbated to the point that my diplopia returned, along with double vision, throat constriction, and blurriness. I also came down with shingles for an entire month, which compromised my immune system. Even though my vision was affecting my daily activities—such as watching TV, using my cell phone, and working—I managed to carry on with the help and support of my family. My husband drove me to my appointments, work (when he could), and errands, and my children picked me up to go out to eat or shop. An optimistic attitude got me through this difficult and frustrating period.

Also, I was taking a proactive approach to finding the right neurologist who I believed had the most experience with treating MG. I solicited recommendations from the MG Foundation of America, NORD, and MG-Muscular Dystrophy Association. My current neurologist's name came up along with his clinical study, and an appointment was scheduled.

January 2019 (age sixty-five) was a pivotal point in my life, as I was looking forward to my first visit to see this new neurologist in my city. He specialized in general neurology, neuromuscular medicine, and neurophysiology along with running an ongoing clinical study. During the initial visit, an MG assessment was performed to confirm my diagnosis, and I was put on pyridostigmine bromide for a three- to four-week period for observation. Surprisingly, this did not change or improve my vision.

I was taken off pyridostigmine bromide and prescribed prednisone for another three to four weeks. This, too, did not alter or correct my double vision. However, it did slightly improve my diplopia.

On the third visit, this neurologist ordered azathioprine along with the prednisone. He went over my treatment and discussed what the next steps would be if I didn't see improvement. Luckily, after two weeks, my double vision and diplopia disappeared. I was so elated to be able to see clearly with minimal blurriness and carry out my daily living skills independently.

So, what's next? It's March 2019, and I'm on a monthly schedule to reduce the prednisone but stay on the azathioprine. Monthly blood work is required for monitoring, and every-other-month doctor visits are required because I am currently in a clinical test study. In summary, I feel blessed that my MG symptoms have greatly improved under the care of my neurologist and anticipate that I will be stabilized and, hopefully, in remission during the next few months.

> *"I was taking a proactive approach to finding the right neurologist...I solicited recommendations from the MG Foundation of America, NORD, and MG-Muscular Dystrophy Association."*

**Expert Comment:**

Any injected foreign protein or recombinant DNA (as is the case with a hepatitis B vaccination) can theoretically trigger the immune system and contribute to the formation of autoimmune disorders like MG. There are case reports, but systemic studies have not confirmed that MG is more common in a vaccinated group than it is in the community. MG is not a contraindication to any vaccination unless the patient has a personal history of reaction to that specific vaccine.

There are certain symptoms that are not typically seen in MG, and their presence should promote a search for other causes, such as brainstem problems, autonomic system disorders, and anxiety. Dizziness, vertigo, disorientation, and foot numbness are not features of MG.

Anxiety is common in myasthenics. The unpredictability of the disease and the vague multiple symptoms may cause it, and prednisone may add to it. What is even worse, symptoms of MG may mimic those of anxiety, and it is not unusual for patients to be dismissed from the ER with anxiety as their diagnosis. Fatigue and hyperventilation with transient blurring of vision are common to both anxiety and MG. These symptoms can also cause diagnostic difficulty when they occur in a myasthenic after remission of the MG, and the clinician will have hard time deciding whether this is a relapse or just anxiety.

The optimal duration of steroid therapy has not been determined. Most clinicians will try to continue the minimal effective maintenance dose for two years, after which they wean the patient off. Probably 25 percent of patients will continue in remission; the rest will relapse within five years, which mandates prednisone at a high dose and not the previous dose the patient was on.

> *"Anxiety is common in myasthenics. The unpredictability of the disease and the vague multiple symptoms may cause it, and prednisone may add to it."*

Shingles is a viral infection that causes a painful rash that usually appear as blisters along the course of intercostal nerves (like a belt around the right or left torso), sometimes on the face, and rarely along other sensory nerves. Shingles is caused by the varicella zoster virus, the same virus that causes chickenpox. After you've had chickenpox, the virus stays inactive in nerve tissue near your spinal cord and brain. Years later, the virus may reactivate as shingles.

The virus may be activated by any factor that lowers immunity, such as stress, cancer, steroids, or chemotherapy. The rash usually resolves within a couple of weeks, but one in five patients (especially the elderly) develop severe lancinating and burning pain along the affected nerve where the skin rash was located. This is called post-herpetic neuralgia (PHN). The pain is chronic and usually requires strong pain medications. Shingles vaccination reduces the risk of shingles and PHN and is recommended after the age of sixty years. I recommend it to my patients at age fifty years.

Prism glasses are very helpful for diplopia. A prism changes the pathway of the light to the eye and aligns the image on the retina. The fluctuation of diplopia in MG makes the prism less effective and less convenient than in fixed diplopia. In patients with purely ocular MG who cannot tolerate medical treatment, a prism may be the most effective and safest method to overcome diplopia. In my experience, when the diplopia becomes more severe, the prism stops working. Hopefully, by then, the patient will be more open to treatment with prednisone.

The patient stated that two weeks after azathioprine (Imuran), the symptoms improved. Azathioprine takes several months to work, and her improvement was most likely due to the steroids, which may take several weeks to work. Patients should be aware of the different duration of onset of action of different medications so that they will remain compliant even if they do not see a benefit initially.

A common problem is lack of response or tolerance to medications. This is even more problematic in patients with negative MG testing. A combination of these two factors make the diagnosis of MG very questionable.

A common cause of interruption of treatment of MG is loss of insurance and lack of affordability. Such an interruption may throw the patient into an MG crisis. Such an unfortunate situation should not be allowed to happen. In our clinic, we inform patients that we will not charge them if they lose insurance and cannot afford a clinic visit. However, we cannot cover the cost of their medications. Pyridostigmine, prednisone, and azathioprine are not expensive, but IVIG and PLEX are.

There are many MG support groups online. Joining these groups may help a patient learn about the disease and coping with it, but they can also increase anxiety.

> *"A common cause of interruption of treatment of MG is loss of insurance and lack of affordability."*

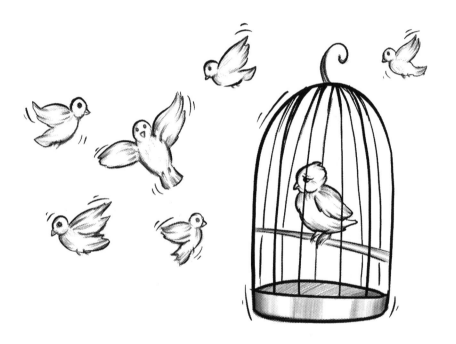

I wish I can go out

# Case #11

## STAYING HOME IS NOT AN OPTION

"I go to a gym regularly to maintain my strength, and I take my medication faithfully, as I want to stay as healthy as possible."

The earliest symptoms began with my facial complexion turning very pale. I had no energy and could not get enough restful sleep. Every time I began to get hot, I noticed I would become very weak in my legs. One morning I awoke to a drooping right eye, and my face looked like I had just had a stroke. A few days later, I could not swallow or eat any food.

The diagnosis began in May of 2018 with lots of blood work being done by my family doctor. He suggested verifying the results with a doctor in my town. Then my wife insisted on making an appointment with her doctor, who is located in a larger city. In July 2018, I was referred to a doctor who specializes in myasthenia gravis. The length of time on the diagnosis was about three weeks.

The symptoms were not easy to cope with because I had only had simple problems in my life. I am only sixty-six, and having to sit in my house all day does not make me happy. I would say it's depression due to not having the strength to walk and function to do your daily chores and activities. So you begin taking it one day at a time and pray you get better.

The first and only treatments I was given were the medications pyridostigmine and prednisone. Some benefits of taking the medication include being able to function more in my daily routine. However, I am still suffering from the side effects of weakness in my legs and my body getting overheated. I have also experienced the side effect of gaining extra weight due to the prednisone. I am still on the prednisone and hope there will be a day when I don't have to take it anymore.

As of today, I am still on the same medications. I did not try to change or alter any medication on my own. I have gone by the dose of medication that the doctor has prescribed for me. But I will admit that the afternoon medication is hard for me to take on a time schedule. Since I have not changed my medication, I have not needed to verify any other medications with my doctor. It would be wonderful to receive a list of over-the-counter and prescription medications that are safe and not safe to take with my current medications.

Myasthenia gravis overall had affected my ability to exercise. I couldn't make one lap around the track. The disease slowed me down in my daily work activities, and since I own a farm, I needed to hire more labor to help me out. To cope with the fatigue, I had to learn to sit down and rest until I could move forward.

I've also experienced difficulty with swallowing. At the beginning, the shock of not being able to swallow was a big concern. I had lost some weight due to not eating but we found that consuming a drink called Boost and eating applesauce, bananas, and soft vegetables kept me functioning. However, after a few months on the medication, I regained my ability to eat again.

> *"I've also experienced difficulty with swallowing...but we found that consuming a drink called Boost and eating applesauce, bananas, and soft vegetables kept me functioning."*

To be honest, my reaction to my diagnosis was a great big surprise. Just reading some of the available information, it was a shock to learn there is no cure, and honestly, it was very heartbreaking. My wife and I are still learning and hope to find out more information so we can take the next steps. As far as my mental health, I try to stay busy to keep a lot of things off my mind.

I hope and pray anyone at the beginning or who has already experienced this disease will receive healing power, great treatment, and a cure for their life. I hope they can be very thankful that they have the strength mentally and physically every day.

**Expert Comment:**

While MG is not a crippling disease and most patients are able to go back to a meaningful level of function, the first three months after the diagnosis can be tough. The symptoms will take several weeks or months to resolve, and medications, especially steroids, can cause depression, fatigue, weight gain, lack of stamina, and exercise intolerance. In addition, some patients have a hard time coping with the diagnosis initially, and they become depressed. Books like this one and support groups can play a crucial role in improving understanding and coping.

> *"MG is not a crippling disease and most patients are able to go back to a meaningful level of function."*

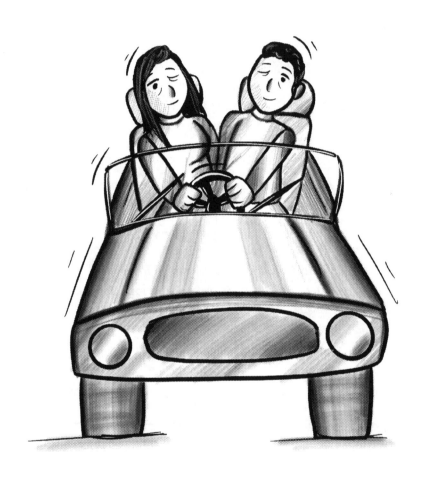

Driving needs two eyes!

# Case #12

## My Brother Got It Too

"Make a list of all your medications and vitamins, keep it updated, and bring it to each doctor you see.

In the spring of 2015, I was on a trip to Savannah, Georgia, with friends. On the last night, we went to a theatrical production where I looked at the stage and realized I was seeing double. I had no idea what caused it and thought it would pass, but it did not. I could see fine up close, but seeing at a distance was a serious problem.

When I got home, I called my regular doctor and got in right away. He thought I might have had a stroke and put me on medication to prevent another stroke from happening. At this time, my left eyelid was starting to droop.

I went to see my ophthalmologist several times, and he did not know what it was. He referred me to a different doctor for a diagnosis. After performing a couple of tests, including a blood test, this doctor diagnosed me with myasthenia gravis. For my treatment, I was referred to a different doctor, one who specialized in MG.

This doctor prescribed the most common medication, and it worked. The double vision ended, as did the eyelid drooping, so my life got back to normal. I could drive and do the things I liked to do. However, I do have periodic episodes of eyelid drooping and difficulties with swallowing. They come and go.

The swallowing issues feel like a muscle spasm, at which time I must stop eating. It will vary in intensity and can be very intense; however, it passes in time. This year, my brother, who is nineteen years younger than me, was also diagnosed with myasthenia gravis. He has had vision, swallowing, and other facial issues as well as fatigue.

For the most part, the myasthenia is manageable, and I live an active life with friends and family. I go to a gym regularly to maintain my strength, and I take my medication faithfully, as I want to stay as healthy as possible.

> *"For the most part, the myasthenia is manageable, and I live an active life."*

**Expert Comment:**

MG may start with double vision to far objects. The images may be oblique, horizontal, or on top of each other, depending on the affected muscles. There are six pairs of muscles that move the eyeballs in different directions in a very coordinated fashion. When one or more muscles gets weak or fatigued easily, the image from one eye will be far away from the image of the other eye. The brain cannot fuse them into one image anymore, hence binocular diplopia (double vision that disappears when one eye is closed) results.

Closing or patching one eye would leave only one image. If a patient complains of double vision even if one eye is closed, then that would not be caused by MG. Such a monocular diplopia may be caused by a disease of the cornea, lens, and retina.

Binocular diplopia can be caused by diseases that affect the nerve of the eyes (from their origin in the brain to their ends in the muscles) and the muscles that move the eyes. Thyroid disease is commonly reflected in the eyes (thyroid eye disease). Patients with Grave's disease (an autoimmune disorder that causes the thyroid gland to be overactive) may present with double vision and protrusion of the eyes (exophthalmos). The muscles are usually thickened and weakened. This condition can be confused with MG, and they both can occur in the same patient.

MG is not a hereditary disease, but susceptibility to it is. Family members of MG patients are four times more likely to have MG than the general population. This may be related to the way the immune system reacts.

> *"Family members of MG patients are four times more likely to have MG than the general population."*

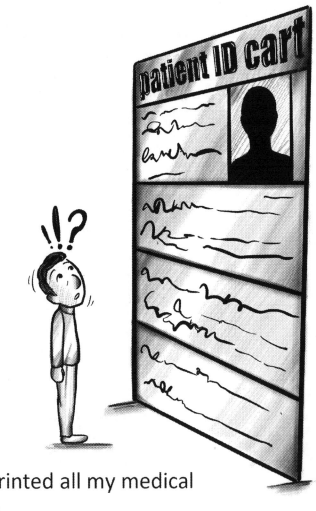

They printed all my medical history.

# Case #13

## CARRY AN ID WITH THE DIAGNOSIS OF MYASTHENIA GRAVIS

"What works for others may not work for you, and you may need to discover your own strategies."

My story started on September 5, 2009. When I woke up that morning, my right eyelid was about 90 percent closed, and I had no control of it. I went to my family doctor and told him how tired I had been lately, and I also showed him my eye problem. He prescribed some medications.

Two weeks later, I was back in his office with no improvement. He put me in the hospital for five days and ran over a dozen tests, including an MRI, CAT scan, daily blood work, and a lumbar puncture. All these tests resulted in no answers, so I was sent to a couple of eye doctors. Again, there were no answers to my problems. I was referred to an ophthalmologist on November 16, 2009, and after numerous tests, he concluded I had myasthenia gravis.

On top of the problems I faced during this ten-week period, I began noticing other symptoms. This included biting my tongue, double vision when moving my eyes left to right, dropping items I was holding without warning, and difficulty swallowing. I had never heard of myasthenia gravis or knew anyone who had it, so I started reading all the information available.

I was sent to see a couple of neurologists, who put me on prednisone and Mestinon. Over the next three and a half months, there was very little improvement, and I was starting to feel the side effects of the prednisone. I was getting very irritable and depressed, and my symptoms were more frequent. It was affecting my job and family interaction.

On March 1, 2010, I was sent to see an MG specialist in the city, and he adjusted my medications by ramping up my prednisone to 80 mg per day and back down to 20 mg every other day over the next few months. I also started taking eight different vitamins. The high doses of prednisone were hard to deal with, as it made me very irritable and I gained lots of weight. It was very hard to go to work and perform my tasks.

A new medicine, Imuran, was added to my daily list in April. At this time, I put together a spreadsheet with all the daily medications and supplements I was taking. Every time I went to see a doctor, I brought this updated list, so in case a new prescription was needed, the doctor could make sure a drug interaction would not take place. I also went to my pharmacist and told him about my MG so he could make sure any new prescriptions would not interact with my current prescriptions.

The last day I was able to work was September 12, 2010. This was a very low point in my life, and it was caused by MG. Not being able to work plus my weakened state of health put me in a state of bad depression. At the time, I thought there was no way out for me. Prayers from family and friends helped with the mental aspect, and the medicine plan my MG specialist placed me on was starting to improve my health slightly.

In late October 2010, a thymectomy was recommended by the specialist. After a few weeks of discussion with my family, I agreed to have it done in December of 2010. The surgery went well, but the recovery over the next couple of months was painful, stressful, and made me question if I had made the right decision.

> **"Carry an ID card that says you have myasthenia gravis, what medications you are taking, your doctor's name, and emergency contacts... This could be lifesaving."**

Three months post-surgery, my overall health was improving a little every week, and by the end of the fourth month, I felt really good. I still have occasional episodes of one or more of the following: biting my tongue, dropping things, trouble swallowing, double vision, or physical weakness (mainly in the afternoon, evening, or after I have been physically active).

However, I can take a Mestinon pill and rest for an hour, and the issues will usually subside. Having the thymectomy was the right decision for me.

Over the past eight years, my condition has remained fairly constant, and so have my medication dosages. I know my limitations, and I have settled in very well living with MG. My symptoms flare up from time to time, but you learn to cope with them by using your medications.

September of this year will mark ten years of living with MG. It has been difficult at times, but nobody said life was easy. Here is a short list of how my life has changed since my MG diagnosis:

- I had to quit working (retiring seven years sooner than I had planned).
- I can no longer mow my yard or work in the flower beds. (I really miss this.)
- I cannot handle outside heat or direct sun for very long.
- My physical limitations far outweigh my can-do list.
- With my weakened immune system, I get ill more frequently, and recovery is longer.
- Most of my activities outside the house are confined to mornings, as by the afternoon, I am fatigued.
- I have had significant weight gain due to prolonged prednisone usage.

Here is a list of suggestions for fellow MG-ers

- Make a list of all your medications and vitamins, keep it updated, and bring it to each doctor you see.
- Consult your pharmacist each time you get a new prescription and bring a current list of medications and vitamins so the pharmacist can make sure your new drug does not have bad interactions with your current medications.
- Find locals in your area with MG, meet with them, and discuss issues and concerns you may have. These folks can have some insight you may not have thought of.
- Keep a positive attitude, and take your prescribed medications as directed.

- Be as active as your current health will let you.
- Carry an ID card that says you have myasthenia gravis, what medications you are taking, your doctor's name, and emergency contacts.

> **"Make an updated list of all your medications and vitamins, and bring it to each doctor you see."**

**Expert Comment:**

This story raises many important points:

- Morning symptoms are not common in MG unless the patient has poor sleep due to sleep apnea or other causes. Symptoms of MG are typically worse as the day progresses. On the other hand, symptoms of stroke are more commonly noticed in the morning due to slowing of heart rate and drop of blood pressure during sleep, which may block a critically narrowed blood vessel.
- Stroke symptoms do not fluctuate but may gradually get better. Droopy eye can be caused by a stroke of the brain stem, cerebral aneurysm, or infarction of the third cranial nerve, especially in diabetics. The latter is associated with severe pain behind the eye and dilatation of the pupil of that eye.
- The most common causes of steroid failure in MG are a low starting dose or premature or fast tapering. There is no universal steroid regimen. A typical dose is 1–2 mg per kilogram body weight of prednisone, and a typical duration is six weeks, followed by a gradual tapering over three months to the minimal effective maintenance dose, which is usually 10–20 mg every other day. Failure to follow this regimen is not common and would mandate verification of the diagnosis and, if verified, addition of a steroid agent in a form of chemotherapy.
- Drug interaction is an important aspect of management. More important is the potential for exacerbating the disease by a

medication. It is advisable that patients inform their physicians about the medications they are using and ask the MG treating physician if they have a question about any new medication they are placed on. Some medications, like metoprolol, have a modest effect and can be continued if needed, but others are absolutely contraindicated, such as streptomycin and quinine. Azathioprine may become toxic if taken with a medication for gout called allopurinol, because they compete on the enzyme that degrades them. Refer to the chart in chapter 9 for drugs to be avoided or monitored in MG.

- Knowing one's physical limitations is an important task that patients should learn. It may require a major change in lifestyle. Both MG and the drugs used to treat it cause fatigue. Mismatch between mental and physical ability may cause depression; keeping a positive attitude and prayer may help. The goal of this book is to enhance coping and to learn about coping strategies from other patients. However, what works for others may not work for you, and you may need to discover your own strategies.

- Carrying an ID informing about the diagnosis and medication is advisable. If you get involved in a car accident and lose consciousness for any reason, the ER physician would avoid giving you medications that may interfere with your MG or drugs used to treat it. If your MG is exacerbated by the accident and you develop a crisis, the physician would know that your respiratory failure is due to MG and would start the right intervention right away. This could be lifesaving.

> **"The most common causes of steroid failure in MG are a low starting dose or premature or fast tapering."**

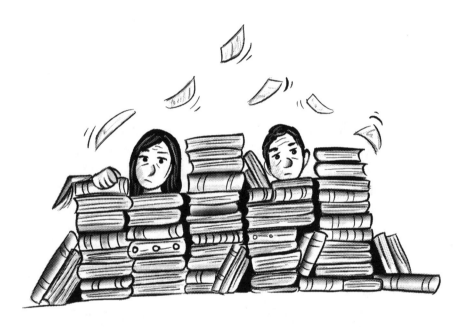

Day 1000, we need a bigger house

# Case #14

## We Choose Not to Give Up

*"First of all, I have never heard of myasthenia gravis.
Did you make that up? What does that mean?"*

Keeping a journal of my husband's journey with myasthenia gravis has helped us stay up to date with his early symptoms and prognosis. We have found our journal to be our biggest asset in dealing with our journey. Why, you ask, *our*? I support my husband wholeheartedly. We go together to each appointment and test. We talk about the way he feels, jot down his/our concerns, list questions to ask before our next appointment, etc. These are a few excerpts from our journal:

- March 6, 2013, my husband experienced his first bout with double vision in his left eye while driving home in the evening from work. This was unusual, so we decided to keep track of recurrences of another episode.
- March 7, his vision was good during the day, but by the late afternoon he had double vision again in his left eye while using new prescription glasses.
- On March 8, his vision was once again fine during the day, however by 9 p.m. he experienced double vision again in the left eye using the new prescription glasses.

- Saturday, March 9, he rested all day. His vision was fine, and he wore his new glasses for very little time.
- He had a few good days with no double vision. Then he had another reoccurrence on March 14 and 15. On both days, he felt pressure/a pulling feeling on his left eye.

We kept a journal through March 21 and decided to go see my husband's primary-care doctor. The doctor then referred us to a neurologist in our hometown. During this time, blood work and a series of tests were done. When results came in, our neurologist suspected what my husband had and then referred us to a neurologist who specialized in neuromuscular disorders for his expertise.

During this initial period, the neurologist here in our hometown also referred us to an ophthalmologist. The use of a prism on my husband's prescription left lens helped with his double vision tremendously. He was able to do work on his laptop and drive back home comfortably.

We acted promptly, and thus our journey with myasthenia gravis began approximately one month from onset with the neuromuscular specialist. We had no idea what to expect and knew nothing about myasthenia gravis. We were very apprehensive on our first visit, but the MG specialist assured us that with proper medication and care, my husband would have a good quality of life. We put our trust in him and thus have traveled this road with our doctor through the good and hard times.

My husband's first treatment was pyridostigmine (Mestinon) 60 mg, one or two tablets every five hours for thirty days for the diplopia. After one month, he was put on prednisone 20 mg four tablets for ninety days. The ninety days turned out to be years. We followed a regimen as outlined by the specialist on a given timeline. Every time we went for a routine checkup, we anxiously waited for the word that my husband would be off this medication. It was a long road, with each dosage logged on a calendar that we kept. We would see this specialist every thirty days at first, then every three months, and now every six months.

My husband is now on 10 mg every other day. What a long journey! The benefit was that this medication worked, although the side effects he experienced were horrendous. His weight gain, restlessness, mood changes, and irritability I would not wish on anyone. My husband turned into someone I didn't know. It hurt to see him go through these changes. On our visit to the doctor, we waited patiently for a change of medication, but it wasn't meant to be.

Along the way, methotrexate 2.5 mg was added. My husband did not have any adverse reaction to the eight tablets taken per week. Blood work taken monthly helps the doctor stay on top of the effects all the medication has on my husband's body. Through prayer and determination, we were adamant to come out ahead. He has been compliant with this plan with me by his side. The MG specialist knew best. We have been fortunate that my husband has not had a thymectomy.

We are vigilant when it comes to medications that may exacerbate MG. We were given a list of drugs that can worsen this condition by our MG doctor. We also know that we can call the doctor's office for verification if need be. We made copies of this list and gave it to our primary-care doctor. Our pharmacist also keeps us informed if there is any conflict. My husband carries a list of medications he is currently taking inside his wallet and car glove compartment. He does this so that if he was to get into an accident, EMS would know which medications to administer and which to avoid.

Myasthenia gravis has affected my husband's daily physical activity somewhat. Even though he continues to do what he has always done, he tends to choose his activities more carefully. If he does something strenuous, he will rest after that. He doesn't push himself to do more than he can. He will rest/relax beforehand, and then he is good to go.

He is fortunate that he does not have swallowing difficulties. Diplopia or relapses have not occurred since the beginning stages documented in our journal. However, we know that pyridostigmine (Mestinon) can be refilled with a call to the specialist. We know that he can rely on the use of a prism on his lens. He has not received IVIG or plasma exchange.

---

> **"Through prayer and determination, we were adamant to come out ahead."**

---

Our world with myasthenia gravis continues. Through our hard work and that of our MG specialist, my husband is now in remission. We can only stress that we all have to be proactive with our health.

Establish an excellent rapport with an open line of communication with your doctor.

We still do not know everything there is to know about this illness. However, we choose not to give up. It is through our MG specialist's knowledge and the insights of others' experiences that we can look forward to a better future in dealing with myasthenia gravis.


**Expert Comment:**

Family support is very important in coping with MG and with the side effects of the medications. The unpredictable nature of the symptoms can cause depression, as patients sometimes do not know what triggers the symptoms. Steroids also may cause depression, anxiety, insomnia, weight gain, and changes in facial features. Having someone who can calm the patient down and understand the behavior is important. Patients can be easily agitated and may become isolated, and that may worsen their depression.

Keeping a journal of the symptoms is very important so that the treating physician will have a clear understanding and the patient will not have to struggle to answer questions about the evolution and nature of the symptoms. Also, the journal will chronicle the symptoms in relation to the effect of medications, which will help the doctor to regulate the dose and frequency of the medication.

There are not many doctors who specialize in MG; therefore, it may be difficult to find a specialist in one's hometown. But it is important that the primary-care physician is aware of the diagnosis and is updated by the treating physician and by the patient about the status of the disease. Communication between the PCP and the treating doctor is crucial, and the patient should ask that medical notes be forwarded to the PCP consistently.

Apprehension is common, especially when the diagnosis is new. It is important that plenty of resources are provided and enough time is given to answer questions and alleviate fears. Establishing a very trustworthy relationship is important. Some patients relocate to different countries for job assignments, and the treating physician should help those patients find a specialist in the new location.

*"Having someone who can calm
the patient down and understand
the behavior is important."*

Mirror, mirror in my hand
Where did my beauty land

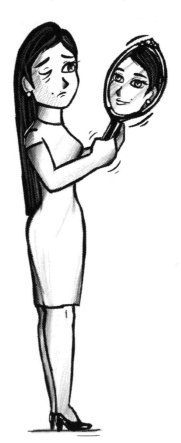

# Case #15

## WHEN YOU ARE A FEMALE

"The lung cancer has now been removed,
and I am currently cancer free."

When you are female, and you are in your fifties … Well, if you are there, you know. Everything is scrutinized every morning. Is there a new wrinkle? Is there something else I need to cover up? Well, I had a magnifying makeup mirror. I did my best to put my best face forward. I had already had a stroke, and it had temporarily taken the feeling from one side of my face. Wonderfully, this had not been visible to anyone else. Praise God.

So, suffice it to say I keep a close eye on my face. At fifty-six years of age, was my left eye drooping? Yes, I thought it was. On my next visit to see my neurologist, I mentioned it. She said that she suspected myasthenia gravis and that the treatment was steroids.

*What?* I thought. *First of all, I have never heard of myasthenia gravis. Did you make that up? What does that mean? I don't want to take steroids. Those are not good. That's all I have ever heard. Steroids are not good. Everyone says steroids are not good.*

"Let's do blood work to make sure," she said. When testing was done, there was no confirmation that I had that confounded disease. Thank God.

Well, maybe it was just age, right? Every day, I looked at my eyes. Was that eyelid drooping more? Maybe, especially in the evening. Now I was having a lot of fatigue, and my legs just would not do what they were supposed to. Going up stairs was getting hard, and walking for exercise was out of the question, because I might not get back. Breathing was getting harder with any exertion, but this was age, wasn't it? Was I that old?

*I'm going to get this eyelid fixed*, I told myself. *I do not have myasthenia gravis, so let's at least look better.* After having more tests to confirm that I did not have the disease, I had the eyelid surgery. It looked great for about a month, and then it drooped again. *What the heck? I give up. I'll live with it.*

Then, on a trip after work to see my family, a change happened. It was dark. I was about an hour and a half into a three-hour drive, and where there was supposed to be only one white line on the right side of the road, I saw *two*. One of the lines was curved, and the other was straight.

I pulled over and considered my options. *I'm halfway to my destination. I have friends at home who may be able to come and get me, but I sure hate to impose on friends to drive all the way out here. My family is still an hour and a half away.* I called, but there was no answer.

The third option was to cover one eye and go on. I chose option number three. By the time I arrived home, I was almost hysterical. It was really frightening. Did I mention I was going somewhere three hours away? Did I mention it was dark? Anyway, I made an appointment for the next day with the eye doctor, who confirmed that my eyes were healthy. *Healthy?* She told me that I needed to see a neuro-ophthalmologist and gave me a referral.

After a day of testing, this new doctor confirmed that I needed to be treated for myasthenia gravis. I was then referred to a specialist in the field. This specialist began treating me three years after I first noticed a problem. He started me on Mestinon, and it worked. My eyelid went up, and I felt stronger for a couple of months. Then I no longer felt it was working as it had been. I was put on a very strong dose of prednisone, and my world completely changed for the better. My eyelid lifted to where it belonged, and my vision came back. My strength returned, and so did my energy. I was able to exercise. The pain I had from arthritis and back pain disappeared.

What a wonderful reprieve from feeling like I was on a downward spiral. Hope! Not all of this good stuff was related to MG, but it was a wonderful break. Of course, I could not stay on that high dose of steroids forever, so some of those symptoms have returned.

Now it has been almost two years, and I am on a much lower dose of prednisone and azathioprine to control my symptoms. I have no eyelid drooping or double vision. Energy-wise, I have learned to spend my energy like I do money: I only have so much. Sometimes I need to rest to recoup so that I can move forward.

All that to say, my life has returned to a normalcy that I can live with. I've made my other physicians aware of my disease and given them the list of meds that make it worse. I also remind them whenever I see them. I still feel uncertain sometimes about my future, as I live alone. I like to plan ahead so that I'm not caught off guard.

When I was not doing so well, I had considered an assisted living environment, and that still may be an option for me now that I'm in my sixties. But now, I do feel like there is no real urgency to make this decision. I have had no side effects so far. I work a full-time job, and I take on as much as I dare. My dream was to go back to Italy, and I did that this year. I'm so glad I did it. I did it. *I did it.*

> **"Having someone who can calm
> the patient down and understand
> the behavior is important."**

**Expert Comment:**

MG affects women at a younger age than men. That is unfortunate. The change in the facial appearance caused by droopy eyelids and the drooping of the corners of the mouth can be devastating. The smile becomes less attractive, and slurred speech is even more socially inconvenient. Steroids have a bad reputation, and ladies are very scared by what they have learned about them.

As a matter of fact, not all steroid side effects occur, and not all patients develop them in the same fashion. Yes, weight gain is common. Reduced carbohydrate intake and increased physical activity tend to counter this problem. Bruises, hair growth, moonlike face, buffalo hump, skin rash, and dilated capillaries can be disfiguring. It is reassuring that most of the side effects resolve when the prednisone dose is reduced. The first few months after the diagnosis are the most difficult ones.

Surgical correction for a droopy eyelid should not be done for two reasons: the first is that the symptom can be treated medically, and the second is that the symptom will return a month or so after surgery if the disease is not treated. Very rarely and in chronic cases, ptosis becomes fixed due to fibrosis of the muscle, and in these cases, surgery may help. Also, one has to differentiate between a droopy eyelid and redundant forehead skin (chalasis), which is common in elderly and can be easily corrected surgically.

A negative blood test is common in ocular MG and should not be used to exclude the diagnosis. As a matter of fact, all tests can be negative in ocular MG, and a trial of steroids may be given to confirm the diagnosis. Positive response occurs in 90 percent of cases. However, one has to be careful, because positive response to steroids is not specific, and other causes of the symptoms should be ruled out with a brain MRI.

> *"Surgical correction for a droopy eyelid should not be done for MG."*

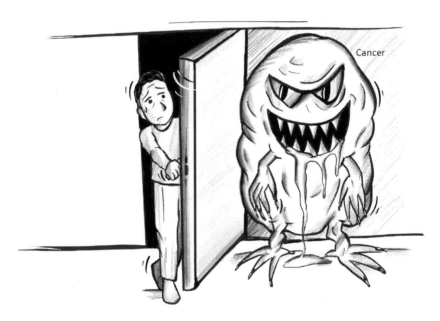

Hello... MG, are you there?

# Case #16

## INCIDENTAL DISCOVERY WAS A BLESSING

In May of 2017, I began to notice I had a drooping eyelid and was having double vision problems. Many vision specialists performed many tests, but none of the specialists could determine the cause of my double vision problem. The last vision specialist I saw recommended that I see this one neurologist who specialized in neuromuscular disorders.

In November of 2017, this neurologist diagnosed me as having myasthenia gravis and recommended I have a CT chest scan. He recommended I begin taking pyridostigmine 60 mg. After about two weeks, my drooping eyelid and double vision problem were corrected without any side effects. About one year later, the double vision problem had not returned, and my vision was great. The CT chest scan that the neurologist recommended was a lifesaver, because it detected a spot on my right lung that was cancer. I could have gone for years and not known I had lung cancer. The lung cancer has now been removed, and I am currently cancer free.

> *"I am cancer free now from a tumor discovered by CAT scan of the chest."*

**Expert Comment:**

Pyridostigmine does not address the actual pathological process of MG as prednisone does. It only makes more chemicals available in the nerve terminal, and it works for four hours. In mild cases of ocular MG, it may be all that is needed to correct the symptoms. It works in about 50 percent of cases. If it works, usually it stops working within a year. However, a minority of lucky patients may sustain improvement for years. I've noticed that most of the long-term responders are elderly. Some patients are very much troubled by side effects like diarrhea, muscle cramps, and excessive salivation and sweating. Adjusting the dose usually lessens these symptoms, and with time, they become more tolerable.

It is not uncommon for patients to be prescribed glasses. Symptoms may be alleviated, but frequent need to change glasses usually alerts the optometrist to the diagnosis, and the optometrist refers the patient to an ophthalmologist. Most eye doctors do not feel comfortable diagnosing MG and therefore refer patients to an eye doctor who specializes in neurological disorders that affect the eyes (neuro-ophthalmologist) or to a neurologist.

A CAT scan of the chest is required for every patient with MG because 10 percent of cases are associated with a tumor of the thymus gland, which is located behind the sternum. Sometimes the scan reveals important incidental findings, such as a lung tumor or thyroid enlargement that will need to be tackled separately. These disorders and their treatment may interfere with MG. They may trigger exacerbation or interfere with symptoms. Their treatment may interfere with the steroids and chemotherapy used to treat MG. An expert is needed to navigate these interactions.

Excessive thyroid function (thyrotoxicosis) is not unusual in MG, as both are autoimmune disorders. This can cause enlargement of the muscles that move the eyes and can be easily detected by ultrasound or CT scan of the orbits. It also causes bulging of the eyes (exophthalmos). However, instead of ptosis, these patients get lid retraction due to increased sensitivity to norepinephrine of the muscles that lift the eyelids.

> **"A CAT scan of the chest is required for every patient with MG."**

I missed the target

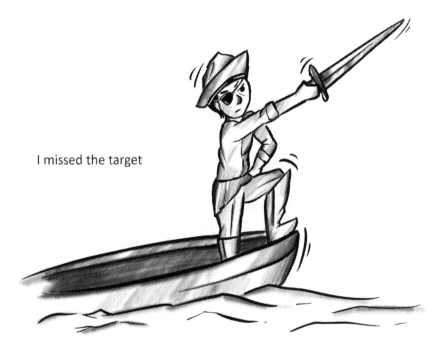

# Case #17

## DIPLOPIA WHILE DRIVING WAS TERRIFYING

In December of 2010, I experienced double vision while I was driving home from work. I had to wear an eye patch for a short period. I could not drive; my wife would drive me and pick me up from work every day for a couple weeks.

I was referred to an ophthalmologist, and her team did extensive tests on my vision. Her thought was that I had myasthenia gravis, and she called a specialist in the field. My wife and I went directly to his office. The specialist examined me, and I was sent for blood work and an MRI. After the results came back, it was confirmed I had MG.

Upon hearing the diagnosis, I was shocked, because I was in my early sixties and had never had any kind of illness or sickness. The first treatment was Mestinon and prednisone 70 mg. The side effects of the medication were an upset stomach and a little diarrhea. The prednisone also made me gain a little weight.

After I stabilized, my MG specialist started reducing my prednisone. When it came to my medication plan, I was always compliant and did not change any dosage unless my physician said to. My doctor then recommended I get a thymectomy, but he could not guarantee that it would cause total remission.

I finally had a thymectomy in December 2012, but only after my wife found a surgeon who would do it with robotic surgery. I had the surgery done on a Friday, went home Saturday, and had my wife drive me to work on Monday. She drove me for a couple of weeks. I do not think I would have had the procedure done if cutting my chest open was my only option. After my operation, my MG specialist prescribed Imuran for antirejection.

After five years of my MG specialist reducing my prednisone, in January 2015, he took me off all medication. Everything was just fine until June 2015, when I had a relapse. My double vision came back. The doctor restarted me again on 70 mg prednisone. I followed his treatment plan, as I still do today.

I've learned that steroids are just a part of having myasthenia gravis, but they have had no long-term effects. Thankfully, I am not on any other medications. My overall health for my age is excellent. Physically, MG does not affect my daily physical activity—just old age is taking care of that, LOL. I do get tired a little more often, but I attribute that to my age. I am seventy-one. I have had no swallowing difficulties with MG, and I have no more diplopia, as long as I continue my medication. I also have not received IVIG or a plasma exchange.

Through this illness, I can't be exposed to excessive heat and sunshine. I realize I will probably be on low-dose prednisone for the rest of my life, and I have no problem dealing with that. Since my MG was ocular, I think being diagnosed earlier kept it from being more severe. If it had been in my lower extremities, I would have brushed it off as just being my age. After having MG for eight years, I have learned to just deal with it.

> **"I had the robotic thymectomy on a Friday, went home Saturday, and had my wife drive me to work on Monday."**

**Expert Comment:**

Thymectomy is indicated in all myasthenics below age seventy when MG is not limited to the eyes. It may take a year and a half for the full effect of thymectomy to appear. It reduces the need for steroids and reduces the number of exacerbations.

MG affects men at a later age. The elderly have slower metabolisms and less tolerance to medications. They need a lower dose of medications. Osteoporosis is more common in the elderly, and steroids increase that risk further. Therefore, it is crucial that calcium 1,000 mg and vitamin D 1,000 units daily are prescribed and a bone density scan is done yearly to detect osteoporosis and treat it. Osteoporosis increases the risk of fractures in the elderly, who are subject to falls. Fracture-related immobility and pain may exacerbate MG. Also, immobility may worsen the loss of muscle mass (sarcopenia) that is common in the elderly.

The elderly tend to be forgetful, and they may forget or confuse their medications. They may need supervision to ensure proper intake of medications. They are more likely to be on multiple medications for other disorders, and it is important to review the list of medications to avoid interaction with the MG drugs.

Also, it is important for elderly patients to have their eyes examined annually to check for cataracts that can be caused by steroids. When the dose of prednisone is reduced, the elderly may develop joint pain, as degenerative joint disease may be masked by steroids. That should not be a factor to keeping them on a high dose of steroids longer, because long-term side effects outweigh benefits. Of course, physicians who treats their arthritis may decide to keep them on a small dose of steroids if appropriate.

> **"Thymectomy is indicated in all myasthenics below age seventy when MG is not limited to the eyes."**

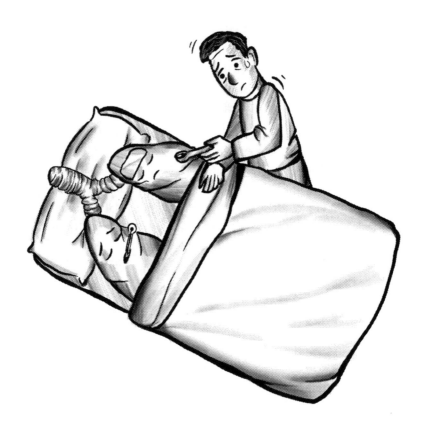

My poor lungs, get well soon

# Case #18

## PNEUMONIA EXACERBATED MY SYMPTOMS

"I think from my first symptoms to the final
diagnosis was about six months."

My diagnosis with myasthenia gravis was made after two or three months, once I saw a doctor who specializes in myasthenia gravis. The doctor knew right away what it was. I had gone to several other doctors before seeing my specialist.

The earliest symptom I experienced was double vision. Coping with the symptom involved having to patch one eye so I could drive. Eating was beginning to hurt my jaw and swallowing was difficult, and I couldn't find ways to cope with it.

When I heard my diagnosis, I was completely shocked. The first treatment I was given was pyridostigmine and prednisone, and I haven't had any side effects so far. Although I experienced weight gain from the steroids, they did help me. My second treatment was a thymectomy. I coped with the surgical stress just fine and didn't experience any side effects. I was always compliant with my medication, and I avoided medication that might have exacerbated my myasthenia by always calling my doctor first before taking anything.

Before being diagnosed, I was seeing double—not side by side but seeing things on top of each other. Then I noticed my chewing and swallowing were affected. I didn't try to exercise, so I'm not sure if my endurance was affected. I coped with the fatigue by working, and I didn't let it bother me.

After the thymectomy, I only had one relapse of symptoms. It was when I got sick with pneumonia and was running a fever. I got a touch of double vision at night, but by the morning, it was gone. The doctor who treated my myasthenia gravis was very attentive, caring, patient, and knowledgeable in his profession.

> *"After the thymectomy, I only had one relapse of symptoms."*

**Expert Comment:**

Fatigue of the chewing muscles is typical for MG. Pain is not. Pain during chewing may be due to inflammation of the temporomandibular joint (TMJ) or, more seriously, inflammation of the blood vessels (vasculitis). There is a condition that usually affects elderly women called *giant cell arteritis* or *temporal arteritis*. Inflammation and obstruction of the blood vessels can cause blindness and stroke. Severe temporal headache, painful chewing, and morning joint stiffness are typical features. This condition should be diagnosed and treated early to avoid grim complications, such as stroke and blindness.

Patients with MG usually have excessive fatigue of the chewing muscles, and they may need to rest during chewing a steak, for example. They may learn how to use their hand to carry their jaw during chewing and talking. Sometimes the jaw remains open (jaw ptosis). Those who cannot open their eyes and close their mouth should be considered myasthenic until proven otherwise.

These cases can be confused with a condition called *dystonia*, when abnormal control of muscle tone is caused by some kind of brain disturbance. These patients usually close their eyes involuntarily and forcefully and periodically, and they may open or clench their jaws and protrude their tongue involuntarily. This confusion is important to recognize, because the botulinum toxin injection used to treat dystonia is absolutely contraindicated in MG, as it slows down further the transmission of impulse from the nerve to the muscle and may trigger crisis.

As a matter of fact, cosmetic botulinum toxin given to the facial muscles may produce ptosis and diplopia after a week or so, which is when the patient does not connect with the injections and fails to mention that to the doctor, and myasthenia is erroneously diagnosed. Fortunately, these cases resolve within 3 months, after the effect of the botulinum toxin goes away. Patients with MG should be alerted that botulinum toxin injections should be avoided at any cost, even for cosmetic reasons.

> *"Patients with MG should be alerted that botulinum toxin injections should be avoided at any cost, even for cosmetic reasons."*

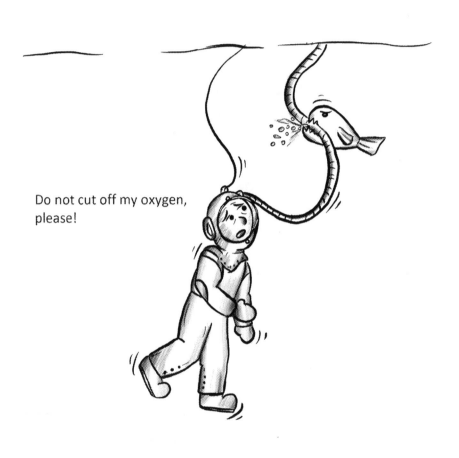

Do not cut off my oxygen, please!

# Case #19

## Suddenly, I Could Not Breathe

"We have a list of medications that patients
diagnosed with MG should not take."

This is my story about myasthenia gravis and how it has affected my life. The earliest symptoms that something was wrong occurred in 2009, but I ignored them. I did not ignore them on purpose, really, but they came shortly after a devastating hurricane, known as Ike, hit our area. My home had been flooded along with my place of employment, and my nighttime job as an adjunct instructor at the local college was affected also.

At this time, I was working at least twelve hours a day helping with recovery efforts due to eight feet of water at the plant where I worked, leaving for a few hours to teach my classes at many temporary locations throughout the campus while cleanup and repair crews were working.

Double vision was my first clue that something was wrong. It was strange to see objects and people one above the other. This did not go away with rest, which I thought it might. I tried squinting, rubbing, and shutting both eyes for extended periods of time. It did not get better, but I soon learned the trick that by shutting one eye, I could see great without the double vision. Time passed quickly due to the long hours at my work, college, and home during the hurricane recovery. We slept in a small travel trailer parked in my driveway, which was difficult to get a good night's sleep in.

Time passed, and it became automatic to close one eye when I drove, worked on my laptop, or even taught a class, so I could function properly. At this time, I still did not know what was wrong, and I just tried to live with it.

When things started to slow a little, I made an appointment with a local optometrist at the mall. When talking to the optometrist, I was completely honest, and he went right to work trying to come up with a prescription for new eyeglasses. I would not have thought it was possible, but with a bunch of prisms and glass, he came up with a prescription where I could see with both of my eyes open. At that moment, I realized this was not right, and there had to be another solution. I continued to work at the plant, teach night classes, and work at home while continuing to close one eye, which allowed me to get by with my daily tasks.

Well, this came to an end one day when the safety representative who worked in the same building as me came to my desk and asked why I had one eye closed. My honest response was that I did it so much, I was not aware I was doing it. He then explained he had noticed it for several days and had decided something must be wrong. He asked me to go to the plant nurse and see what she said.

The plant doctor happened to be there that day and had noticed I was asking a lot of questions. He decided that it was in my best interest to go home, because he felt I had experienced a stroke and needed medical attention. So that day, one employee drove me home, and another drove my auto home.

> **"Time passed, and it became automatic to close one eye when I drove."**

First was a trip to my family MD, who thought the situation was very strange and that it might be best to go back to the optometrist. I disagreed, so he suggested that maybe a neurologist would help. At that point, I was thinking my doctor thought my symptoms were just in my head. However, I agreed to go.

Several weeks later, I went to see the local neurologist. The neurologist did a variety of tests over several visits, including eye charts. I am not sure what he found with those tests, but he finally decided I needed a blood test.

I quickly agreed. I'd had many blood tests in the past, but this time was different. They actually came to my house and drew a few vials of blood, which were sent immediately to a laboratory in Boston, Massachusetts. I kept thinking about how much this test would cost me, because at this time, I was at home from work on short-term disability.

My neurologist called me to come into the office, so I did. He then explained that he had run two tests, and both were positive for myasthenia gravis. Well, of course, I had never heard of this disease, and I was shocked when I learned MG was an autoimmune disease. I was afraid of the unknown, and it really took me off guard.

I think from my first symptoms to the final diagnosis was about six months. My neurologist recommended that I go see a doctor who was much more familiar with this disease than he was. So arrangements were made for me to see a doctor who specialized in MG.

I was nervous at this time, and being the researcher that I am, I went straight to my PC to read all I could on the disease. There were multiple stories written by patients, so I tried to read all of them in just a few weeks. Most of the medical terms and explanations were not so clear to me, other than the fact that it was a type of autoimmune disease and had many symptoms, some being worse than others.

When I visited my new doctor, he explained the treatment I would be going through and that it would take some time to get better. In other words, I would not get better overnight. The big medicine turned out to be one of the most common medications, known as prednisone, which I was going to be taking large doses of. Those who have taken this drug know that it will cause you to put on weight, and I was no exception. There were some other drugs that I took at very precise amounts and times alongside the prednisone. It seemed very soon after treatments that my double vision got better, and I was getting around pretty good and felt okay.

> **"I was afraid of the unknown, and it really took me off guard."**

The side effect was about 60 pounds of weight increase. Some of that was my fault, due to not working and being at home every day. I was always hungry, and everyone seemed to bring me a great dish of food to enjoy. I continued to get better, and soon the massive amounts of steroids were being decreased a little every few months. At this time, everything was going as expected, and I was happy I was getting better.

Unfortunately, a bad incident that was entirely my fault happened next. I had been on a reduced amount of steroids, and during the holiday, I ran out of pills. I did not refill the prescription because I had an upcoming appointment in a few weeks, and I thought he might reduce my amount even more.

What happened next is very hard to explain, but almost out of nowhere, I started to have extreme difficulty with breathing. I continued to get worse, and it was getting to the point where I was becoming scared. I contacted my doctor, and he asked me to get to the ER hospital in the city so he could come in to treat me. We were instructed not to go to the local ER, for they would not treat me correctly. I needed to travel to the hospital in the city where he was located.

I called my wife, who was at work, and told her about what my doctor had instructed me to do. She immediately left work to pick me up and take me to the hospital. When I tried to get in my wife's car, I quickly found out that I could not catch my breath once I sat down. It was getting worse, and I was having a hard time catching my breath. This was such a scary situation; I realized I needed to stand up in order to get the air I needed.

I tried several times to get in the car for the two-hour trip to the hospital, but I was not successful. I then had the idea to use my CPAP machine to get me the additional air needed. After a short time, I was able to sit down with the mask in place and let the CPAP do its job and allow me to sit and breathe at the same time.

My wife communicated to the doctor that there was no way I could make the trip. He called in a prescription for the large doses of prednisone that were needed to start my treatment from the beginning again. The procedure worked, and soon I could breathe on my own again without the CPAP. Patients must take their medications following their prescription instructions each day and never deviate.

Thymectomy surgery was discussed, and I even talked to a surgeon who agreed to remove the thymus gland. I also talked to my heart doctor, who did not think it was worth the risk to open me up. This is because I had already, years earlier, had a heart valve replaced. He explained that a chest can only be opened up a few times before other complications can occur, so I chose not to remove my thymus.

We have a list of medications that patients diagnosed with MG should not take. One time, I was prescribed a medication by the ER that should not have been administered. Luckily, my wife was alert enough to catch this, which was good, because I might not have caught it.

During the worst parts, I did not feel like exercising, and that added to my weight gain. I got through this and joined the local gym. I found out due to knee and hip problems that the only thing I could do was ride a bike, so sometimes I rode the bike up to five to six miles at a time. Now that the MG is in remission, I can do just about anything—no muscle weakness, no double vision, and no other reason I can't enjoy life and work some jobs. Currently, I continue to watch my weight and continue with my teaching job at the local college, as well as enjoy my family and friends.

> **"Now that the MG is in remission,
> I can do just about anything."**

**Expert Comment:**

It is not unusual for MG symptoms to appear for the first time during or after stress. This may include a hurricane, car accident, emotional upset, a viral illness like flu, pregnancy, delivery, or bad news. By the same token, exacerbation and crisis may be triggered by stress. Symptoms may progress quickly and should not be taken lightly, especially shortness of breath. Patients should not drive to the ER. Calling 911 would be safer. An ambulance is equipped to deal with severe shortness of breath that may require oxygen.

Symptoms of MG may develop gradually and intermittently, and diagnosis may be delayed. Diplopia can be mild initially, and patients learn to avoid it with an eye patch or closing one eye. Eye closure can cause mild frontal headache. Squinting and rubbing do not help; closing eyes and rest usually do help, but for a short period of time. Changing glasses and prisms usually help, but again, for a short period of time.

Double vision can lead to accidents. Images can be on top of or beside of each other or oblique. In severe cases, the eyes deviate abnormally and become crossed. In more severe cases, patients have to turn their heads to see to the side because the eyes do not move at all.

Sometimes, symptoms mimic a stroke, such as ptosis, diplopia, and slurring of speech. MRI of the brain may reveal incidental changes that are common in the elderly but may be erroneously interpreted as consistent with stroke. Patients are placed on aspirin and dismissed. Symptoms may disappear as a part of the fluctuating nature of the disease, enforcing the diagnosis of stroke until symptoms come back and prompt another look.

It is not unusual that patients do not refill their medications after symptoms resolve, or they may think that if there are no refills ordered, the medications were intended for a short period of time. This usually triggers a relapse, which may take the form of a crisis. When symptoms return, the patient has to start steroids at a high dose as in the beginning, which is contrary to the common belief that the previous dose would be enough.

> **"It is not unusual for MG symptoms to appear for the first time during or after stress."**

Hello Karen, is this your twin?

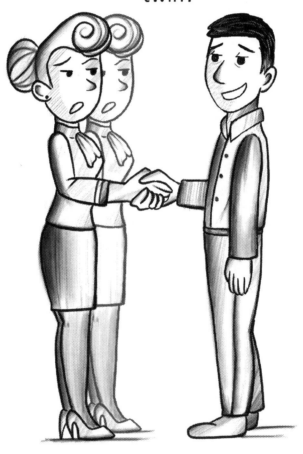

# Case #20

## I Was Diagnosed with Ocular Nerve Palsy

My friends have often said that I have two speeds—
either full speed or stop—and I guess that would
be a good description of my lifestyle.

My earliest symptoms of the disease appeared about a week after I had total knee replacement surgery. Supposedly, the surgery or the impending death of a close family member caused the stress that allowed the disease to appear. My right eye began to droop about a week after my knee replacement, and shortly afterward, I developed double vision (diplopia). A trip to the ER and an injection of antibiotics confirmed the start of my difficult journey toward a diagnosis.

Five days later, I had a visit with my ophthalmologist, who diagnosed me with third nerve palsy. Two days later, my speech was impeded, and swallowing became very difficult. The swallowing difficulty caused a weight loss of twenty pounds in a two- to three-week time period. During that time, I had to eat very slowly and drink liquids to sustain myself.

As a result, another trip to the ER was in order, with a CAT scan and an MRI performed. Naturally, the doctors were thinking blood clot or stroke symptoms due to the surgery. Diagnosis: some type of palsy.

The next day, I followed up with a visit to my family doctor. He was not satisfied with the palsy diagnosis and referred me to a neurologist. The neurologist performed a blood test, and as he suspected, I was diagnosed with myasthenia gravis. Like most people, I had never heard of this autoimmune disease and was surprised at how serious the disease could be if not treated properly and correctly.

My first treatment was a boost of steroid injections to alleviate the symptoms. Unfortunately, that was not very effective, and a stronger injection was prescribed. It worked, and the symptoms eased. Of course, with the steroids came anxiety, irritability, and sleeplessness. I was given additional medication in a pill form of pyridostigmine (Mestinon) and prednisone. The previously described side effects continued, with additional leg cramping at night and hand cramping during the day, especially when performing repetitive tasks with my hands. I feel the Mestinon was the culprit for the cramps.

I was referred to an MG specialist, and according to him, the Mestinon only masked the disease. So I decided to take myself off the Mestinon, and the majority of the cramping disappeared. Currently, under the care of this doctor, I am on a higher dose of prednisone for six weeks and then a steady reduction for another period of time. I have not had any other treatments or procedures (thymectomy, IVIG, or plasma exchanges). I have a list of medications to avoid, and I have discussed them with my doctor.

Because of fatigue, MG does affect my daily physical activity. I can still perform my daily tasks, but I have to approach them at a slower pace. By pacing myself and periodic resting, I have been able to complete my activities without much difficulty. I did have a slight relapse with the diplopia when my previous doctor reduced my medications. My MG doctor prescribed a higher dose of prednisone, and as a result, the diplopia symptoms have subsided.

Psychologically, MG has affected my life, but I try to overcome it by not dwelling on it and by coping with the reality that there is no cure. Hopefully, I can achieve my goal to reduce or stop the intake of steroids and improve the prognosis for my long-term health.

> **"I had a visit with my ophthalmologist, who diagnosed me with third nerve palsy."**

**Expert Comment:**

Double vision due to MG can be caused by weakness of one or more of the six muscles that move each eye in different directions. Such a weakness, if isolated, may be misinterpreted as paralysis of one of the three nerves that supply the eye muscles—in this case, the third cranial nerve. Other symptoms, such as swallowing or speech difficulty, would not be consistent with isolated nerve palsy. Also, fluctuation of symptoms is typically seen in MG and not in the other conditions.

Swallowing difficulty starts mild and with liquids only, and may progress to severe and affect all kinds of food consistencies. Coughing and choking frequently lead to reduced oral intake and loss of weight, and sometimes aspiration pneumonia, which would worsen the associated breathing difficulty. Swallowing difficulty should not be taken lightly, especially if it occurs with breathing difficulty.

> *"Swallowing difficulty should not be taken lightly."*

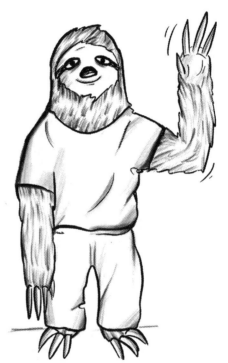

Didn't you know that sleep makes you happy?

# Case #21

## KEEP POSITIVE ATTITUDES AND SLEEP WELL

I would pray and sing praise music, which also seemed to help.

As far as family records go, there is no history of myasthenia gravis on my mother's or father's side of the family. However, in 1940, my father began to have problems that included coughing, choking, and increased salivation. Because he had trouble eating, he began to lose weight and was sent to San Angelo in 1942 to a sanitarium (this is what the continuing care facility was called at that time). However, they were unable to diagnose him with anything but acute bronchitis there.

In 1943, he came back home by ambulance, and I remember my oldest sister Katherine and I were waiting for him outside. He was bedridden from that time until his death in early 1945. Although his bed was elevated to help him breathe, he was very cheerful and alert. Due to his symptoms, my family and I feel that he probably had myasthenia gravis.

I graduated from high school in 1955 and was married in June of that same year. My first son was born in 1957 and my second in 1961. At the time, I was working part-time at General Telephone in Baytown.

I began working for Sears in July of 1961 as a switchboard operator. I worked there for a short time until an automated system was installed. I then worked in sales and soon became a division manager in Softline's departments for three years, as well as a manager and decorator consultant in both drapery and carpet. It was a job in which I had to visit homes, carry heavy samples, and do a lot of reaching and stretching to measure windows. I went through a difficult divorce in 1983; however, both of my sons were married, so it was not as traumatic as some are.

In late 1983, I met the love of my life, and we were married in 1984. I worked until late 1987, and around that time I began to have headaches and loss of strength. We thought they were caused by some compressed disks in my neck, so I had surgery, thinking that was causing them. However, my condition was no better, and because of this, I went on long-term disability.

At this time, I went to several doctors to try to find the problem. In 1991, I went to the hospital to see a doctor who had been recommended by my pastor's wife, who was suffering from some neurological problems. This doctor treated me with intravenous gamma globulin and a thymectomy. As he diagnosed me with myasthenia gravis, I asked him what that was and how to spell it.

I saw him very often that first year due to tests and treatments. He prescribed the drug Mestinon (pyridostigmine) for me. In the years, ahead, insurance companies tried multiple times to give me the generic version, but it always caused me great weakness and regression. I know that in the United States, the drug is very expensive, and the alternative drugs from Mexico and other countries did not work for me. I called Canada and was able to purchase the drug from the same pharmacy that has supplied my Mestinon for years at an affordable price. I continued to order my medicine from there for almost twenty years.

My friends have often said that I have two speeds—either full speed or stop—and I guess that would be a good description of my lifestyle. My husband and I worked together after his retirement to restore two lovely homes in two different cities in our state. My tasks were mostly designer, gopher, painter, and arranger. My husband, however, was very good at whatever he did.

> **"The drug is very expensive, and the alternative drugs from Mexico and other countries did not work for me."**

We were always active in our local church and in mission work that needed to be done. God called us both to serve as volunteer missionaries. We served our local church the first year, he as building coordinator and I as a volunteer secretary.

In 2003, we called a friend at one of the mission centers in our city to ask if she had anything that two old people could do. She was delighted to have us and wanted us to serve as house parents to the summer missionaries (college students ages eighteen to twenty-four). We felt like fish out of water the first year but settled in and continued to serve in that capacity until 2016. We were both having some health problems. My husband had spent that last year on oxygen 24/7 for his COPD, and I was having some atrial fibrillation issues.

My husband went to his heavenly home in 2017. My sons and I did not feel that it would be safe for me to live in the city I resided in, as it was about a four-hour drive away from their jobs and homes. My youngest son was divorced and had a home with a pool and pool house. So he doubled the size of the pool house so that I could live in his backyard. It was easy to care for and has worked out well for me. I have furnished it with things from my old town so that it feels like home. My personal belongings and some of my furniture fit into the bungalow (as we call the pool house) nicely.

I have missed my friends and my home, as we had lived in the previous town for twenty years. But, as stress is not good at all for an MG patient, I want to be calm in my lifestyle. I am trying to involve myself in activities in the new town. I also want to spend more time with my other son and his family, as well as with the five grandchildren and four great-grandchildren in the area.

My first priority has been seeking healthcare providers in the nearby metropolitan area. An MD in my new area set up appointments for a cardiologist in the bayside and another doctor in the larger metropolitan area. My neurologist is doing tests and researching my physical conditions.

I feel good most days and try to live a normal life. I have learned that some rest time is very necessary each day. I try to keep one full day each week clear for down time. The only thing that interferes with this is my insomnia. I go to bed at an early or reasonable hour, but I usually wake once or twice during the night. When I was diagnosed with myasthenia gravis, I was given a 180 mg Mestinon that was time-release, and it worked to give me a good night's sleep. I seem to need six to eight hours of sleep in order to feel my best.

I would encourage anyone diagnosed with myasthenia gravis to keep a positive attitude, stay busy, and depend upon the Lord for strength in order to make life more meaningful.

> *I would encourage anyone diagnosed with myasthenia gravis to keep a positive attitude.*

**Expert Comment:**

Myasthenia gravis medications can be expensive. Pyridostigmine and prednisone are usually not. However, pyridostigmine timespan 180 mg (long-acting) is not easily obtainable in the United States; patients usually get it from Mexico or Canada. IVIG is expensive, and it is hard for uninsured patients to pay for it. If they are admitted through the ER for MG crisis, then IVIG or plasmapheresis will most likely be used regardless of the insurance.

With age, there is a change in the way the body handles drugs. The metabolism slows down, and getting rid of the medicine becomes less effective; therefore, the medicine may accumulate in the blood, causing more side effects. As a general rule, I start with a lower dose in the elderly (older than seventy years), and if patients are already on medications, as they grow older, I would try to reduce the dose by half. Also, the elderly are more likely to develop drug interactions because they are usually on multiple medications. Periodic review of their medications list by their neurologist is important.

Lifestyle changes very often occur as people get older. In addition to age-related restrictions, the elderly need more rest and frequent naps to restore energy and overcome fatigue. They are encouraged to be involved in social activities and to remain active mentally and physically, but they should know their limitations.

Insomnia exacerbates fatigue and should be treated as much as possible. Prednisone causes insomnia and should be taken in the morning. Some medications for insomnia may worsen fatigue, such as anticholinergic and antihistamine, and they are nor recommended in MG. Zolpidem tartrate is usually recommended in a dose of 5 mg at bedtime.

A positive attitude has healing properties in MG even more than other diseases, as fatigue is partly psychological.

> *"Elderly are more likely to develop drug interactions."*

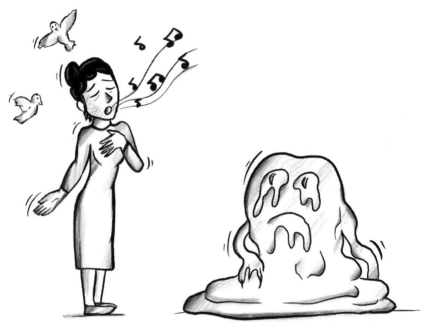

Stop it. Your voice is anti-myasthenic

# Case #22

## PRAY AND SING PRAISE MUSIC

Rest is for the dead.

I began experiencing occasional double vision (diplopia) last May. At first, I didn't think much of it, but it gradually became more frequent. It got to the point where I began to be concerned with my ability to drive safely. I could always cope by closing one eye, but that was stressful and limited peripheral vision.

My difficulties were compounded when I was selected for a jury in the last week of June, which lasted two months. Now, instead of a relaxed retirement lifestyle, I needed to be driving to and from downtown through rush hour traffic each day. Riding the bus was not an option. The eight a.m. to five p.m. court schedule made scheduling doctor appointments a challenge.

The diplopia became more frequent, but I found that it helped to stay well hydrated. I would stop at a Burger King before entering the freeway on my way home from court and get a large lemonade. I would pray and sing praise music, which also seemed to help.

> **"Slurring of speech was embarrassing at work."**

In July, during the trial, I began to experience other symptoms. The muscles in my cheeks would become very weak, to the point that it became difficult to hold food in my mouth when chewing. I began to occasionally have slurred speech. This was embarrassing to experience in front of the other jurors. A phone conversation with my family doctor, followed by an appointment during a break in the trial, seemed to indicate that I wasn't having strokes. The best guess was that it might be some kind of migraine.

After the trial ended, I saw two ophthalmologists, the second of whom was able to diagnose the myasthenia gravis and refer me to a doctor who specialized in the field. But, by the time the multiple appointments with the ophthalmologists were scheduled and blood work done, it was mid-November, and I had begun to experience a notable loss of strength in my arms and fatigue in my legs when I walked any significant distance. It would occasionally be difficult to hold my head erect.

The doctor prescribed a daily dose of prednisone and provided pyridostigmine to be taken as needed. The effects were impressive and immediate. Within a couple of days, the weakness in my mouth and slurred speech had disappeared, and they have not recurred. The diplopia and weakness in my arms and neck would recur, but they were not as bad and seemed easy to control with the pyridostigmine. After several weeks, I've been able to cut back on the pyridostigmine to almost nothing without much problem. But it's good to know that it's available if needed, especially when I need to drive in heavy traffic or do anything strenuous.

It's now mid-January. The doctor has me on a schedule to reduce the prednisone. We haven't yet scheduled a thymectomy. I've been following the instructions he gave for the medications. I appreciate the flexibility he gave with the pyridostigmine, to take one or two every four to six hours as needed. I haven't yet come to the point of having any second treatments or relapses.

I had lost ten pounds before I started the prednisone. I assume this was because of the way the MG made it difficult to eat. I gained that back and more after starting the medicine and enjoying the Thanksgiving/Christmas holiday season. I'm now trying to cut back and get the weight back down.

Aside from taking a ballroom dancing class with my daughter, I don't have a regularly scheduled exercise program. I'm not sure how to approach that. I instinctively try to avoid pushing the exercise to the point that I feel limited by the MG. I like to feel that I have reserve capacity available. But perhaps that's not the way I should be thinking about it.

Psychologically, I haven't felt any strong emotions. The whole thing was an unwelcome surprise, but as medical issues go, it could be much worse. The medicines seem to be effective. I haven't yet had to make any profound changes to my lifestyle. As a retired person, I have the option of sleeping late or being as lazy as I want to be. But I don't want to live that way. I try to keep to a reasonable schedule: get to bed on time, wake up and get dressed on time, make a to-do list, and execute it. Myasthenia can cause a feeling of weariness that can tempt me to sit and vegetate. But I'll keep putting one foot in front of the other. I'll get all the rest I truly need, and then as I start moving out, the weariness seems to dissipate.

> *"Within a couple of days, the weakness in my mouth and the slurred speech had disappeared."*

**Expert Comment:**

Since the main characteristic of myasthenia gravis is fatigability, one has to avoid repetitive activities like prolonged talking and chewing. Rest is usually refreshing. Jury duty would be tiring and is not recommended. Most judges understand and honor a physician's recommendation for exemption.

Sometimes the muscles that hold the head up are affected as a part of progression of the disease or even in isolation and become the presenting symptom (dropped head). Usually, history will reveal double vision, but when not, other possibilities, such as muscle inflammation and Lou Gehrig's disease, should be excluded. This symptom may become crippling as the patient cannot hold his or her head to look forward. Some patients use their hands to lift their head or use a device to hold their head. Pain in the back of the neck is common.

There is a condition that usually occurs in the elderly called *isolated neck extensor myopathy* (INEM) that can be confused with MG. This is due to degeneration of the paraspinal muscles due to age and is much less responsive to treatment than MG.

> *"Some patients lift their heads with their hands to be able to see."*

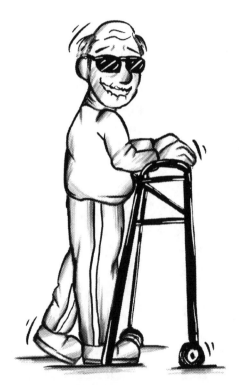

Hey bro, check out my moves

# Case #23

## EIGHTY-SEVEN YEARS OLD, AND FUNCTIONING

In January of 2009, I began having symptoms of droopy eyelids, difficulty with walking and swallowing, and weakness in the knees and chest. I first sought out my ophthalmologist, who repaired my eyelids. Months later, my eyelid continued to drastically droop. So, I went for another consultation, and I was finally referred to a neurologist. In January 2010, I was diagnosed with myasthenia gravis.

I began IVIG treatments along with oral steroids. My symptoms did not improve after one year of treatment. In January 2011, I was referred to a doctor who specialized in MG. Once I became his patient, I learned so much more about this disease. My doctor and his staff were always patient and understanding of the countless questions I had concerning my treatment and my condition. The central line I had was replaced with a fistula after a few months of receiving plasma exchange treatments. In the beginning, I had weekly treatments, and they eventually became biweekly.

At eighty-seven years, old, I continue with plasma exchange. The treatments have kept my condition from worsening. While receiving treatments every three weeks, I remain able to get around with a walker or cane. Although the treatments have not been a cure for me, they have allowed me to continue functioning.

I appreciate my doctors and all their staff for such great care. Their patience, kindness, and positive demeanor keep me going.

> **"The plasma exchange have kept my
> condition from worsening."**

## Expert Comment:

About 5 percent of patients with MG do not respond to pyridostigmine, prednisone, azathioprine, mycophenolate, and IVIG. Some develop limiting side effects, such as a drop in the blood count from chemotherapy, severe diabetes and hypertension, stomach bleeding from steroids, and kidney failure or leg-vein thrombosis from IVIG. At least half of these patients respond to plasma exchange. This modality is normally reserved for MG crisis, and it is temporizing, but sometimes it is used as a chronic therapy.

Frequency varies. Sometimes it works for one week only, while other times it is needed every three months. Instead of puncturing a vein and an artery every time, it is very convenient in these cases to insert an AV shunt similar to the one used for the renal dialysis patients. The shunt may be place in an arm or a leg. Occasionally, the shunt gets obstructed. This can be treated with a clot-dissolving medicine locally or by mechanical dilatation.

Surgical repair of the eyelids in MG is not a good idea, because droopiness almost always returns. It is wise for these patients to be cleared by a neurologist first. If permanent causes of droopy eyelids are found, then surgery may be an option. There are three major causes for droopy eyelids besides MG. A form of muscular dystrophy called *oculopharyngeal muscular dystrophy* that is associated with swallowing difficulty and runs in families usually does not cause double vision. Chronic progressive external ophthalmoplegia is another condition that causes progressive loss of the ability to move the eyes and droopy eyelids. Sometimes retinal degeneration and heart block occur as well. There is also a form of myasthenia that is congenital, and it occurs during childhood (congenital myasthenic syndrome).

None of these conditions respond to the classical treatment of myasthenia. The latter one may respond slightly to pyridostigmine. Also, fluctuation of the droopiness of the eyelids is not a feature of any of these conditions.

> *The plastic surgeon… immediately suspected MG and administered an ice pack test, which opened the eyelid.*

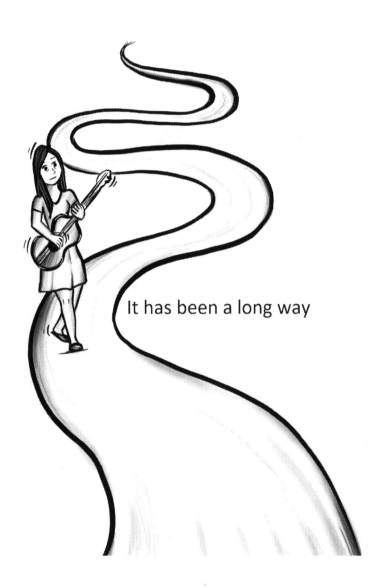

It has been a long way

# Case #24

## ROAD TO DISCOVERY

It made me reflect on the fragility of life and the
need to be flexible in my plans for retirement...

"I'm not sick, but something is wrong."

These are the words I said to my husband that started our quest to find out just what was wrong. I suppose the symptoms could have been developing for quite some time before they began to impact my life.

At seventy-three or seventy-four, I was still playing a pretty good game of doubles tennis two or three times a week. One day, I just could not make my feet move to react to a ball. It just flew past me, and I watched it without being able to stick my arm and racket out or move my feet to go toward the ball. I also began to notice at about that time that my eyes were not reacting as normal. They would not make the normal adjustment from far to close or vice versa.

I have always had quite good eyesight, and I have always been thankful and appreciative of this gift of sight. I just decided that maybe age was catching up with me. This began my journey with my eye doctor that lasted about a year. Bless him, each time I returned, my sight was different. After several prescriptions, I finally gave up on glasses helping me.

About this time, some friends and my husband and I were going out to Arizona for a hiking trip. I found at times I would be quite shaky, and other times I did okay. But I definitely knew that I needed to rest daily to be able to participate. This was not my normal MO. I used to have a quote on my refrigerator that said, "Rest is for the dead." Again, was age catching up to me?

Having become quite tired and worn out from hiking, I was having trouble chewing and also noticed I would drool while chewing. I slept most of the two-day drive home from Arizona, and this was when I said, "I'm not sick, but something is wrong."

My primary-care physician thought he knew what might be wrong but wanted me to see a rheumatologist. That doctor did extensive testing and blood work and eventually said he felt I needed to see a neurologist. I was seen by a bright young neurologist who put me through some physical testing and then began asking about the symptoms that were troubling me. I described my changing eyesight, weakness in my legs and arms (I was having difficulty holding my arms above my head while doing my hair), chewing, and drooling. Finally, I said, "And sometimes I can't whistle."

She said, "I know what is wrong. I studied this in medical school. You are the classic case of myasthenia gravis."

Whew … a reason for all of this with a *name*! My immediate question was, "Is this progressive?"

She said, "Maybe not, as we have found it early, but I do want you to see an endocrinologist to check your thymus. Sometimes there is a problem in the thymus, and with surgery, this can be cleared up." Alas, the thymus was not the cause for me.

I was put on a medication called pyridostigmine bromide. It is a pretty uncomplicated medicine with relatively few side effects that does not damage internal organs. It does not accumulate in your system and seems to last four to six hours. It was discovered during the building of the Panama Canal as a cure for malaria, but apparently helped MG patients as well.

> *"My doctor said now I was going to have to learn the "art" of managing my pill usage."*

I began taking this medication immediately, and it started to work quite quickly. I began at half a pill four times a day. My doctor said now I was going to have to learn the "art" of managing my pill usage. I have learned that it actually *is* an art. I have since cut back to three times a day, and it seems to be working just fine. There are times when I get a bit shaky, so I take another half a pill.

My one side effect is that it seems to cause eye twitching. Dropping back to three times a day has helped curb the twitching. I feel I have a good grasp of managing my MG. I still like to rest in the afternoons, but often I just take some time out and read for a while.

Myasthenia gravis is not a common condition. Most doctors know its name from their medical studies, but because it affects such a small number of people, it is not easily diagnosed. I feel very blessed to have been diagnosed in a relatively short period of time—about two years. I do not have pain, and I am gradually adding activities back into my life. I hope to return to the tennis court and feel, at almost seventy-eight, that I am doing very well. I count my blessings every day.

I have met some amazing and wonderful and compassionate professionals along the way and feel fortunate to live in this wonderful country during this time of medicine that can help so many people live a productive life with a little or a lot of help.

I thank all of these great people who have guided me and ultimately helped me find the answers. I also thank my precious husband, who made me his total focus to discover the problem. He continues to this day to be my best friend, best supporter, and cheerleader.

I thank you one and all for your guidance and knowledge.

> *"My husband was my biggest supporter, friend, and cheer leader."*

**Expert Comment:**

The road to discovery is usually long, especially if the symptoms are mild. Fluctuation of the symptoms and resolution with rest delays seeking medical advice. In younger age groups, symptoms may be attributed to psychological causes. On the other hand, onset can be severe, and in those cases, diagnosis is made within a short period of time. A typical scenario is that an optometrist who notices frequent change of eyeglasses and abnormal fatigability of the eyelids and double vision refers the patient to an ophthalmologist or neuro-ophthalmologist who then makes the diagnosis.

Frequency and dosage of pyridostigmine may be calibrated according to need. It usually works for four to six hours. Sometimes a tablet (60 mg) is enough, while other times two tablets are needed at a time. Muscle twitching and diarrhea can be limiting, especially in the elderly. Some physicians prescribe prolonged-acting pyridostigmine that works for twelve hours. Sometimes pyridostigmine is used around the clock instead of "when needed." These decisions are made by the treating physicians according to the patient's needs.

> *"Unlike prednisone, pyridostigmine can only be taken when needed."*

> *"Fluoroquinolones such as ciprofloxacin are also associated with worsening of symptoms of MG."*

A happy house 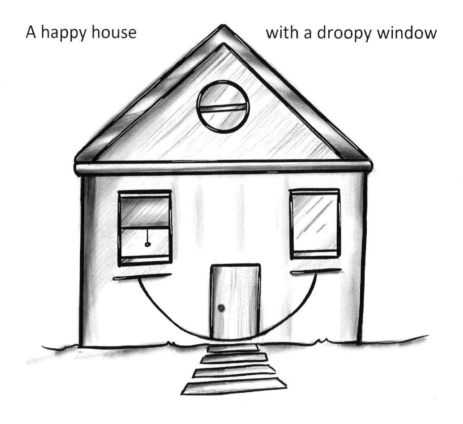 with a droopy window

# Case #25

## TAKE IT DAY BY DAY

"I have had to let people help me more than usual, which has been hard for an independent person."

On a Sunday evening, after a pleasant day of playing golf, I looked in the mirror and my right eyelid was drooping. My first reaction was that I got an insect bite on the golf course or something similar and that it would go away. On Tuesday morning, it was still there, so I walked into my ophthalmologist's office. My usual doctor was not at that location on Tuesday, so I saw another doctor who could not see an insect bite or anything wrong with the eye itself. He suggested I see an ocular plastic surgeon. The next available appointment was the following Monday. The first doctor did not identify that I had a neurological problem or mention myasthenia gravis.

The plastic surgeon at the ophthalmology clinic immediately suspected MG and administered an ice pack test, which opened the eyelid. We also had a long conversation about the role of diet, focused on organic and keto, a favorite topic of his. He then referred me to the neuro-ophthalmologist, who could see me the next day.

Actually, I saw an MG specialist at another time who also did an ice pack test and ordered a blood test to check for MG antibodies. Basically, the diagnosis was confirmed two weeks after first onset when I was back in her office.

All I had was an eye droop; no double vision, since I was only seeing

173

with my left eye. There was slight weakness but no interference with daily function. I was also very tired and ready to go to bed by seven-thirty or eight o'clock and then sleep ten to twelve hours.

I continued to work at my full-time job but stopped evening activities because of fatigue. By four in the afternoon, I was ready to go home and rest. Luckily, my work allows me to set my own hours.

I brought my wife along to hear the diagnosis. She was familiar with MG because Aristotle Onassis and Roger Smith, Ann Margaret's husband, both had it. She kept me calm, saying that I just needed to tape up my eyelid and keep going. My wife and I both have research backgrounds, so we hit the internet to learn everything we could. We decided we both needed to modify our lifestyles to include organic eating. I needed to lose weight so I could position myself to reduce the blood pressure medication I had been on for twenty-five years plus other medications from my primary-care physician, urologist, nephrologist, and so on.

This all came as a shock, coming out of nowhere on a day where I had felt healthy, happy, and had a pretty good game of golf. It made me reflect on the fragility of life and the need to be flexible in my plans for retirement and business succession. I was well informed of the possibility of systemic exacerbation but just blocked that out of my thinking.

My first treatment involved increasing doses of Mestinon, going up to 4 × 60 during the day and 1 × 180 ER at bedtime. The left eye opened halfway, rarely all the way, and sometimes slid shut. I was having severe nighttime leg cramps from the Mestinon, which woke me up in pain. I experienced severe abdominal cramping during the day, with itching rashes over my legs and back. This went on for about six months. All in all, it was not really satisfactory.

> **"We were familiar with MG because
> Aristotle Onassis and Roger Smith, Ann
> Margaret's husband, both had it."**

During that period, I consulted with a nutritionist who suggested a dietary approach to MG. My wife has been wonderful at cooking special meals during all this. I lost twenty-five pounds, and my blood pressure has come down considerably.

On a Monday afternoon, I was sitting at my office desk. My right eye was down three-quarters of the way, and then the left eyelid went down. Both eyes were down! Panic! I got myself home after calling the doctor's office and getting the first appointment the next morning. My doctor said it was time to see the MG expert. Thursday, I saw the MG specialist, who prescribed prednisone, which I started the next morning.

I'm four weeks into the prednisone, and both eyes are open. Not only am I not tired but I'm also energized and sleeping six hours a night instead of ten. I wake up with energy, focused and organized, like I'm Bradley Cooper in the movie *Limitless*. Perhaps I'm *too* energized; I felt over caffeinated the first couple of weeks, but that has calmed down.

I hadn't been able to read more than five pages in a book without falling asleep. The second weekend on prednisone, I read two full five-hundred-page books, played golf, went to the movies, cleaned up around the house, and generally acted like the Energizer Bunny. My rashes cleared up. I had no more cramping. My arthritic knee felt better. My inflamed gums improved. It was great stuff!

When the prednisone opened the right eyelid, it took a little while for the two eyes to work together on distance vision. Now they are coordinated, and I can see much more sharply than before. Another steroid benefit.

It wasn't all perfect. The Mestinon was causing leg cramps that were interrupting my sleep. I was concerned the lack of sleep was affecting my work performance, so I cut back on the Mestinon. I had started on the generic and then ordered brand name to see if it made a difference. I was poorer, since the brand name was outrageously expensive, but no change in results. My advice is to take the generic.

When it comes to other medications, all my doctors have the MG Foundation list. My cardiologist didn't care and didn't want me to change my beta-blocker and calcium channel blocker. Therefore, I am in the process of switching doctors. Working with my PCP, I moved to minimal doses of Cozaar and Norvasc for my hypertension, but with my weight loss, my readings have dropped twenty to thirty points. I have also reduced going to restaurants, and I am eating at home more, where my wife prepares wonderful low- or no-sodium meals.

I needed antibiotics for periodontal work and took amoxicillin, which I tolerated well, even though I always thought I had a penicillin allergy.

My MG specialist said that was probably a reaction to the preservative in injectable penicillin, and I should be able to take the pills, which was correct. So I've had a full course of both antibiotics and steroids. I feel very cleaned out.

I've concluded that certain doctors only care about their area of responsibility; they don't care if the MG is systemic as long as I don't have a stroke or a heart attack. I had a stent after a blockage in 2005, so I know I need statins and blood thinners, but I think I can do a lot for blood pressure with diet and exercise. I dropped furosemide, K-Dur, allopurinol, and alfuzosin to reduce my overall level of medication. I was taking one medication to make me pee and another to stop me from peeing. Crazy. I've concluded I've been way overmedicated and had a long talk with my PCP about a philosophy of minimizing medication.

At this moment, seven months into my MG adventure, I feel terrific physically and grateful mentally for every good day that I am having. I know the next test will be when I work off the prednisone, but I really don't think about that. I just think about how good I feel today. I do feel thankful that I live in a city with a wonderful medical community. I am also thankful that at sixty-eight years old, I have Medicare and supplemental insurance that has basically covered the cost with the exception of the brand-name Mestinon.

I hope that telling my story in detail will help others.

> *"The second weekend on prednisone, I read two full five hundred-page books."*

**Expert Comment:**

Double vision requires vision in both eyes. If one eyelid is completely droopy, double vision will not happen. That is the case if one eye is blind for any reason.

Generic pyridostigmine is not much different from the brand. However, some patients insist that they feel better with the brand, and they are willing to pay the difference.

If MG patients need antibiotics for any reason, they should alert the prescribing physician about the diagnosis, since some antibiotics may affect MG adversely. Aminoglycosides like neomycin, streptomycin, and amikacin are contraindicated. Fluoroquinolones such as ciprofloxacin are also associated with worsening of symptoms of MG. Beta-blockers and calcium channel blockers are not absolutely contraindicated, and if the patient has been taking them for a while and they are working, they do not have to be discontinued. I would avoid starting a patient with MG on them in particular; there are many alternatives.

> *"If MG patients need antibiotics for any reason, they should alert the prescribing physician about the diagnosis."*

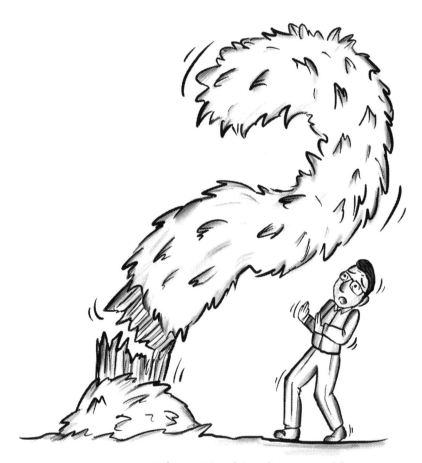

What Kind is this tree!?

# Case #26

## A Disease I Had Never Heard of Before

The symptoms started with double vision while I was driving. A few days later, I went to the ophthalmologist, which led to a strabismus specialist. Both doctors asked if I'd had a stroke. After this, my blood pressure was elevated for about two weeks, causing me to need changes in my blood pressure medication.

The strabismus specialist wanted an MRI of the brain and specific lab work. They prepared a pair of glasses for me so I would be able to drive. While waiting for the results of the tests, I began having difficulty chewing and swallowing. It reminded me of TMJ (which I have a mouthpiece for).

After I had the MRI of the brain and the lab workup, the specialist identified the problem as myasthenia gravis, a disease I had never heard of before in my life. From the strabismus specialist, I was referred to a neuromuscular disorders specialist for further workup. This whole process occurred from August 21 to October 31.

The specialist prescribed pyridostigmine 60 mg three times a day. After taking the first one or two tablets, I experienced massive nonstop diarrhea with stomach cramps. After notifying the office, the doctor suggested taking half the pill (30 mg) three times a day with Imodium. Within two weeks of starting the medication, the double vision disappeared, and the diarrhea lessened with the Imodium. After several weeks, the Imodium could finally be decreased. I am currently taking the Imodium about every three days while on the 30 mg three times a day of pyridostigmine.

With myasthenia gravis, my symptoms included difficulty swallowing as well as occasional difficulty while chewing. I am aware of the trouble I have with the muscles in my mouth, so I eat slowly, and I order softer types of food. I know that when the difficulty with chewing and swallowing starts, it will temporarily go away, but it does make me anxious.

Additionally, you cannot take this medication without eating or drinking a substantial amount of food, which can be difficult when you're not hungry. The type of food I intake with the medication could have direct consequences and result in diarrhea and abdominal cramps. First, I use milk to help coat my stomach, and then I take half of the tablet midway through food intake. In the morning, I eat oatmeal and drink milk. Some days work better than others; even if I follow the same pattern, it may work differently. Nevertheless, the medication is extremely important. Regardless of the complications, I still need to take the medication.

I am tired by late midday. I have had some very good days and some not-so-good days. I never changed the medication on my own without talking with the doctor's office. It is important to review your medication list with your doctor. One of the medications I am on (atenolol) had to be reduced due to the possibility that it would exacerbate the myasthenia gravis. I had a CT scan of my chest to determine if there was a tumor in my thymus, which there was not. The fatigue happens daily. I have learned to rest (usually watching television) and then in about two or three hours, I feel better.

Regarding mental health, this has been difficult. The medicine must be taken with food three times a day, and it keeps you extremely aware that there is a problem that is not going to go away, and you must schedule your day around it. I am not used to being tired in the afternoon and having to sit and rest. I have had to let people help me more than usual, which has been hard for an independent person.

I am very aware of the benefits of staying on this medication, and that makes it worth working through and staying with the schedule on a daily basis. To be aware is a good thing.

> **"I am not used to being tired in the afternoon and having to sit and rest."**

**Expert Comment:**

Pyridostigmine is a medication that has been around since 1955. It blocks the enzyme that breaks down the acetylcholine—the chemical that is needed for muscle contraction. Therefore, it increases the availability of the ACh in the nerve muscle junction. It starts working after forty-five minutes and lasts four to six hours. Side effects are common and include the following:

- diarrhea
- nausea
- vomiting
- abdominal cramps
- increased salivation
- excessive eye tearing
- increased bronchial secretions
- constricted pupils
- facial flushing due to vasodilation
- erectile dysfunction

Most of the side effects improve with reducing the dose and frequency. Diarrhea is minimized by Imodium to be taken an hour before pyridostigmine.

> *"Most of the side effects of pyridostigmine will improve with reducing the dose and frequency."*

I shall heal you now.

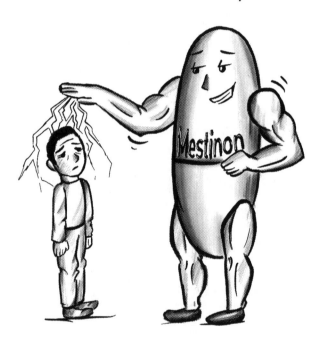

# Case #27

## You Can Still Live a Full Life

"Some 20 percent of cases go into spontaneous remission..."

My earliest symptoms are easy to describe. I can identify their appearance almost to the hour. I was flying from Texas to Florida on July 9, 2004. I had a connecting flight in Texas, and my first flight was late, leaving me with thirty-five minutes to make my connection. We landed at the farthest gate in B terminal, and my flight was at the farthest gate in E terminal, which is about a mile. I literally ran the whole way.

When I boarded my flight and sat down, I looked out the window. The white line on the tarmac had a curved line running off it to the left. That was the beginning of the diplopia, which later was diagnosed as myasthenia gravis. I had no other symptoms, even though at first, I was concerned that the stress had caused me to have a mild stroke.

It took until November to diagnose what had happened. I went to my regular doctor, who thought I had impacted sinuses from golfing in the dry summer heat. Her medication did no good, so I then tried my ENT, who thought it was caused by a bad allergy attack. Nothing he did worked either.

A friend of mine who is a doctor recommended his ophthalmologist. The ophthalmologist determined I had a brain tumor. With that, I went to my wife's hospital, where she got me into both an ophthalmologist and a neurologist. By then, my eyelids had started drooping, and the doctors concluded I had third nerve paralysis. I don't remember any treatment from them.

When I got back to Florida, a colleague suggested his ophthalmologist, who had solved a similar problem for him. This doctor took a look, sent me for an MRI, and diagnosed me on the spot. He then sent me to a neurologist who took one look and said I was classic myasthenia. He prescribed Mestinon, which cleared up the vision problem. By January, I was going into remission, but I kept the Mestinon handy for flare-ups.

Before I was prescribed Mestinon, I had great difficulty driving and dealing with my work because of the blurry and double vision. I was determined that this would not hinder my daily life and was actually relieved when I got the diagnosis because now there was something that could be done. The Mestinon cleared up the vision. At first, I took it four times a day, then slowly reduced to only when I had a vision problem. I had no other symptoms, so it was an issue that I easily dealt with.

I had no other treatment until 2007, when I had a more severe flare-up. I had to learn to distinguish between blurred vision caused by my myasthenia and blurred vision caused by my allergies. I had one occasion where I mistook an allergy attack for myasthenia and took Mestinon. It took several hours for the resulting effect of blurred vision to wear off.

In June of 2007, my wife and I were on a trip through Europe. We had been in Germany, Belgium, and France, and I began to notice I was getting blurry vision again. We had an apartment in Cambridge and had planned a trip to the Our Lady of Walsingham Shrine, which is the Lourdes of England. I went to a healing service and was anointed with water from the holy well, and my vision cleared up. I have never had the vision issue since.

However, in August, we were with some friends in Florida, and I noticed my speech was slurred. We went out to dinner, and I realized I had great difficulty swallowing. Because of the vision issue in Europe, I had made an appointment with a myasthenia gravis specialist for when we got back. By then, I really needed the appointment. The specialist examined me and prescribed 80 mg of prednisone daily, which we tapered off as I improved. The prednisone slowly sent me into remission, and we reduced it to 10 mg until 2014. The side effects on the high dosage sent my blood sugar out of control, and I still stay on Janumet (medication containing metformin and sitagliptin) to keep it stable.

I have kept to the prednisone regimen faithfully since 2007, but in May of 2014 we decided to reduce the dosage to 5 mg every other day. In June, I was in Italy and noticed that when I held my camera with one hand, I got shaky very quickly. I had no other symptoms. In September, however, I was conducting a church service, and as it progressed, my speech got increasingly slurred. By the evening, I could not swallow. We upped my dosage to 70 mg per day along with Mestinon and began the tapering again. Today I am on 7.5 mg every other day. There are no plans to try reducing it again.

I am very careful about other medications that may exacerbate the disease. My original neurologist gave me a list of things to avoid, so I check any over-the-counter drug very carefully for contents. I warn any doctor to watch for contraindications in medications. I have had one bad experience with an antibiotic that was so new that my ENT did not know the side effects. I took one capsule and thought it affected my eyes. The next day, when I took the second, I realized my speech was getting funny. I checked the information from the pharmacy and saw the first note that said not to prescribe it for myasthenia gravis patients. It is now red-flagged in my ENT's office.

When the disease is active, I cannot exercise. The 2014 episode was so bad I could not even stand from a sitting position without being lifted. In remission, there are still effects. From the ocular experience in 2004, I have never totally recovered my depth perception, especially when looking down. I find that I tire much more easily than I ever did before, but I know some of that is being eighty years old. I have learned that when I tire, I need to stop and rest. I think part of my last two episodes was the result of rushing to catch trains, lifting luggage, and tiring myself. I have learned to pace myself while still carrying on an active life and schedule.

The difficulty swallowing was perhaps the most difficult thing to manage. I had to learn to take very small bites of food and chew them almost to a paste. In both events, I found that there was a spot in my throat that was less affected, so I made sure to try to swallow at that point. That took some careful thinking with each bite. Even so, I lost about fifteen pounds each time. It is not a diet I recommend.

While this is not a disease I would wish on anyone, my experience is that it is manageable. I recommend that anyone who has this diagnosis learn as much about the disease, its effects, and how to live with it as possible. Knowing that there are others who have the disease and live full lives makes it much easier to accept and go on with life.

> **"While this is not a disease I would wish on anyone, my experience is that it is manageable."**

**Expert Comment:**

There are many medications that can worsen symptoms of MG or even trigger a relapse that can be unpredictably severe. Sometimes patients do not correlate the worsening with the culprit drug. It is important to go over the medication list for every patient with MG, especially at the time of exacerbation. The following list of commonly used drugs should be kept accessible at all times:

- **Fluoroquinolones** (e.g., ciprofloxacin, moxifloxacin and levofloxacin): These are broad-spectrum antibiotics that are associated with worsening MG. The US FDA designated a black box warning for these agents in MG in 2011 due to the reporting of thirty-seven cases of patients whose symptoms worsened. Eleven of them needed artificial ventilation and two died.
- **Macrolides**: This is a class of antibiotics, such as erythromycin and azithromycin (Z-pack), that may exacerbate myasthenia. Their use should be monitored for worsening symptoms. They do not carry a black box warning. One of the members of a related class (Telithromycin) was associated with a black box warning, and it has been withdrawn from the market because of liver toxicity.
- **Aminoglycosides**: A class of antibiotics like neomycin, streptomycin, gentamicin, kanamycin, tobramycin, and amikacin used to treat tuberculosis and resistant gram negative infections such as endocarditis, these may trigger severe MG crisis even if used in a form of eye drops.
- **Botulinum toxin**: This is used to treat certain neurological disorders, such as dystonia, hemifacial spasms, and blepharospasms, although

it is more commonly used cosmetically for facial wrinkles. It works by preventing the release of acetylcholine from the nerve terminal. In MG, the receptors where this chemical works are already blocked, and preventing its release can be catastrophic. As a matter of fact, even non-myasthenic patients may develop symptoms of MG-like double vision and ptosis after botulinum toxin injections. The effect usually appears a week after the injection and lasts for three months.

- **Corticosteroids**: It is paradoxical that the most effective drug for treatment of MG is associated with worsening of the symptoms in 10 percent of cases within the first two weeks of initiation. If the disease is severe enough, such worsening may lead to respiratory compromise. This side effect should always be explained to the patient so that initial worsening would not lead to interruption of the medication. If the symptoms are severe, patients may need to be admitted to the hospital for treatment with IVIG or plasmapheresis.

- **Beta-blockers**: Commonly prescribed for hypertension, heart disease, and migraine, beta-blockers may worsen MG. Use with caution. However, patients should not panic when they find out that they have been on a beta-blocker like metoprolol or atenolol for a long time despite being myasthenics. If these medications have been effective in treating a cardiovascular condition, they do not have to be discontinued. We do not recommend that treatment with these agents be initiated in someone with MG, however.

- **Magnesium**: It is used for eclampsia during pregnancy intravenously but should only be used with extreme caution in myasthenics.

- **Drugs used to treat disturbances of the heart rhythm**: Drugs such as procainamide, quinidine, and mexilitenine are relatively contraindicated due to the potential for worsening MG. Use with caution.

> *"Beware that prednisone may worsen your symptoms before improving them."*

- **Statins**: Drugs like atorvastatin, pravastatin, rosuvastatin, and simvastatin are used to reduce serum cholesterol but may worsen or precipitate MG. Use cautiously if indicated and at the lowest dose needed. It is not practical or scientific to stop these medications or not to use them, as they have been shown to be effective in reducing the risk of stroke and heart attack. They are more commonly associated with muscle cramps and muscle disease.

- **Hydroxychloroquine (Plaquenil)**: Used for malaria, rheumatoid arthritis, Sjogren's syndrome, and lupus, this medication may worsen or precipitate MG. Use with caution.

> *"I wish I had started on the*
> *medication even sooner, because it*
> *worked and really did help me."*

- **Checkpoint inhibitors**: This new class of medications—such as pembrolizumab (Keytruda), nivolumab (Opdivo), and atezolizumab (Tecentriq)—used to treat cancer can not only exacerbate but also cause MG. Like statins, they can also cause muscle damage.

Regarding the impact of faith on healing: Complementary and alternative medicine (CAM) have become popular, and diseases like MG can be a fertile ground for it. The unpredictability of the symptoms and the frequency of spontaneous remission in MG are factors that enforce the spread of holistic approaches. Some 20 percent of cases go into spontaneous remission, and if this is preceded by taking an herbal medicine or going to a worship place or being exposed to a form of faith healing, then an association would be made. When the disease relapses and a CAM approach does not work, patients seek medical advice without questioning the logic behind the first improvement.

There is no well-designed, placebo-controlled study to show the superiority of acupuncture, herbs, or any holistic or CAM approach over medical treatment. Ironically, there is no placebo-controlled trial demonstrating the superior effect of steroids either, but for a different reason. Steroid testing has become unethical because of the clear lifesaving effect that has been experienced over decades.

It is hoped that the claims about certain herbs will be investigated systematically. After all, many medications are derived from plants, such as physostigmine (the precursor of pyridostigmine), atropin, digoxin, and morphin. There are several thousand herbs classified in China as medically useful, but clinical trials are scarce. The same applies to acupuncture. It is not safe to use any of these methods to replace standard medical therapy (what is known in China as Western medicine). However, unless there is a specific reason not to, CAM, including faith healing, can play a positive role as an adjunct approach in alleviating anxiety and fatigue, an important component of the disease.

Since stress can trigger an exacerbation, it makes sense that fighting stress would induce remission, but can that factor alone control the disease safely? I do not know. There is no scientific evidence to support this. There is no evidence against it either. Practically, there are patients who fail with CAM approaches but respond to steroids. I have not seen patients fail with steroids but respond to CAM. For the sake of this article, CAM includes:

- acupuncture
- aromatherapy
- biofeedback
- chiropractic medicine
- diet and nutrition therapy
- herbalism
- holistic nursing
- homeopathy
- hypnosis
- massage therapy
- meditation
- reflexology
- spiritual healing
- traditional Chinese medicine (TCM)
- yoga

> *"The unpredictability of the symptoms and the frequency of spontaneous remission in MG are factors that enforce the spread of holistic approaches."*

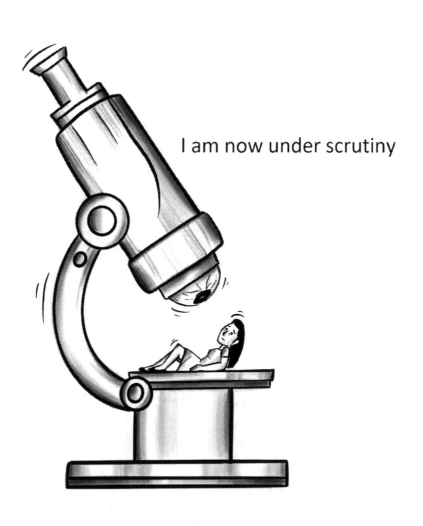

I am now under scrutiny

# Case #28

## I Was Not Used to People Always Staring at Me

In 2010, I was leaving a restaurant I had just ate at. While I was driving, I was looking to turn, and I noticed the traffic looked like it had doubled. I also noticed the same problem when I drove by the plate glass windows of a building. Pictures hanging on the walls would be slanted, and when I would look at myself in the mirror, the image appeared distorted. It's very difficult to explain. I noticed the images were doubled there too, and I knew then that something was wrong.

I saw several regular doctors who referred me to other doctors. No one could figure out what was wrong, I had lab tests done, and I even had an eye doctor perform tests on my eyes, but nothing was indicated. I was eventually referred to a doctor who specializes in disorders like myasthenia gravis.

I had a lot of difficulty coping with the double vision, especially when I was driving. More specifically, I had a lot of difficulty trying to get down a curb. The problem was that I would see too much shadowing from the trees, so to help me, I would either cover one eye or close it while I was driving.

Over time, before my diagnosis, my symptoms began to worsen, and my eyelid drooping was worsening. It had become so obvious that when I went out to eat, people would stare at me. By this point, I had gotten used to dealing with the double vision, but I was not used to the people always staring. When I was finally diagnosed with myasthenia gravis, I felt relieved that I finally had an answer to what was going on with me—that someone had finally found something.

I started on a large amount of prednisone. Eventually, over time, I was tapered off of it and put on azathioprine, I think. But I had to get put back on the prednisone again. I have to say that all the medication does help. The prednisone really helps me, but it is hard because sometimes, when I get back on it, I get the moon face.

One of the medications I had side effects with was the azathioprine. I didn't know I was allergic to the medication, and I ended up in the ER at one point because I looked like a duck, I was so swollen. Instead of getting off the medication, I adjusted to it, and I was fine for a time. However, when I was eventually taken off the medication and put back on it, I experienced bad side effects again, so the medication was switched to a different one.

Sometimes I have to go back to my doctor when I have taken a lot of antibiotics of a specific kind, because that will cause me to have a relapse of symptoms. When this happens, I always go back to my physician, and he adjusts the medication accordingly so we can get my symptoms under control. I am always compliant with the medication given by the doctor, and I have never tried to change it on my own.

The only time myasthenia affects my physical activity is when I have a relapse of symptoms. When I have a relapse, I see cars floating and all sorts of things. It is very irritating, but other than that, it does not affect my ability to perform physical activities.

I have now gotten used to myasthenia, but when it first started occurring, it was hard to adjust because it was so strange. I would see doors and cabinets crooked, and cars looked like they were stacked on top of one another. Some looked like they were floating. At first, this could take a toll on you mentally. It was difficult, because this was happening before I was diagnosed, so I was trying to overcome it, but I didn't know what was happening or how much worse I was going to get because it seemed like it was getting worse at the time. These questions made the situation even scarier than it was, because the situation was already kind of weird. I was thinking it was just going to get worse.

I wish I had started on the medication even sooner, because it worked and really did help me. Once I started taking it, I felt back to normal.

> *"It had become so obvious that when I went
> out to eat, people would stare at me."*

**Expert Comment:**

Symptoms of MG are as worrisome to friends and family members and coworkers as they are to the patient. Over the phone, speaking for more than a few minutes leads to slurring of speech, and people may think that the patient is drunk. Trouble swallowing and chewing gets worse as dinner goes on, and people may think something is wrong, but they cannot tell what it is. Stroke is often suspected, but symptoms resolve with rest, and the patient does not want to see a doctor until the symptoms become persistent or impairing. Distortion of vision can go for a long time before the diagnosis. Driving in the evening becomes hard due to poor eye adjustment to oncoming headlights.

> *"Driving in the evening becomes hard due to
> poor eye adjustment to oncoming headlights."*

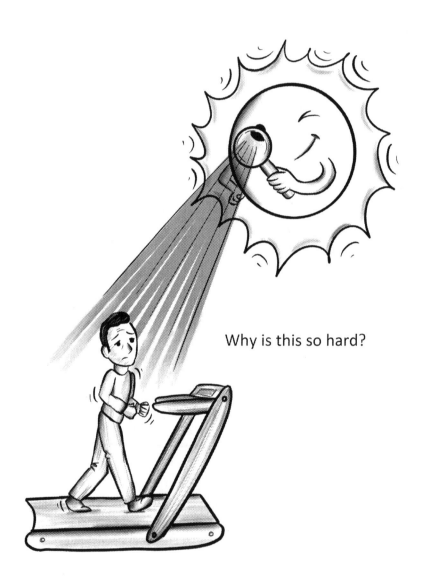

Why is this so hard?

# Case #29

## STAY AWAY FROM HEAT AND STRESS

"The first six months after the diagnosis are probably the hardest."

I was first diagnosed with myasthenia gravis in 2012. It started with a drooping eyelid and then double vision. My wife noticed my drooping eyelid. I tried to brush it off by saying I was tired and overworked, but then I started having blurry vision, and at times I could not even see the food on my plate. There were times when my vision was so bad I could not drive, because I could not see well enough.

I first went to a local eye doctor, and he thought the droopy eyelid was a cosmetic issue and referred me to a neuro-ophthalmologist. That doctor did some tests and referred me to a neurologist. The total time before I was diagnosed was around five to six months. It took a while, because there was a time when I was in denial, and then it took some time getting an appointment, and then the doctor had to run tests, evaluate me, and diagnose it.

> *"The total time before I was diagnosed
> was around five to six months."*

My first reaction to my diagnosis was sadness and disbelief, but then I was a little relieved that my neurologist knew what was going on with me, because I was at my wits' end living with this condition. It was so hard;

195

I don't know how I was able to go to work and act like I could function normally. There were times when the blurred and double vision were so concerning. I had to put everything in the hands of my faith and my doctor.

My first treatment was a very high dose of a medication called prednisone. I was prescribed 80 mg daily. The dose was so high that the pharmacists had to double check before they would even fill it. The medication affected me strongly and very quickly. Weight gain, mood swings, depression, and tremors were just a few of the side effects. I would have outbursts; this affected my life and my family's lifestyle. I would scream at my wife for no reason. I could not control my emotions. I could not sleep or relax, and I questioned whether my reaction to the medication was worse than my actual condition. I was also placed on other medications, all of which had additional side effects.

I have had ups and downs, remission, and three relapses of MG. The relapses were due to work conditions and altering of the dosage of the medication by my neurologist. Every time I thought we were on a good path toward dealing with my condition, I would have a setback and would have to start over on the high dosage of prednisone again.

Heat, stress, and tiredness affect my condition instantly. I cannot mow our yard like I have always done. I hire someone to mow our yard in the hot summer months and in the fall. In the winter, I can do it, but I have to keep stopping to take breaks. I cannot function like I used to. Chores, errands, and normal types of work tire me so much more easily. I used to love staying busy at home, but now I am limited, and I cannot function at the pace I used to.

I have read so much literature regarding my condition, and it scares me. I can only go by what my life is like now, not by the literature. My body is not like it used to be. It's not a matter of aging, it's what this condition has done to my nervous system and to my body.

I had a very good job and made very good money, but because of this condition and how it has affected me, I have been forced to retire earlier than planned. I have followed my doctor's plan for my treatment. I go for regularly scheduled office visits, and I have never altered the dosage unless my doctor has instructed me to do so. I am thankful that we found a doctor who has helped me, and my family is grateful for the wonderful care from him and his office staff.

> **"I have read so much literature regarding my condition, and it scares me."**

**Expert Comment:**

*Snowflake disease* is another name for MG because it differs so much from person to person. The degree of muscle weakness and the muscles that are affected vary greatly from patient to patient and from time to time. Not only that, but factors that may trigger a dormant disease or worsen symptoms vary greatly. The following are documented triggers:

- **Physical stress and overexertion**, especially repetitive activity
- **Stress associated with major surgery**, which may require a higher dose of prednisone to combat. If the adrenal gland is suppressed for a long time by chronic steroid use, it may not be able to produce the needed dose of cortisol during stress, leading to adrenal crisis, which is manifested by low blood pressure and vomiting. That is why we try to taper prednisone to every other day so that in the days off prednisone, the adrenal will produce its own and it does not atrophy. It is important for the surgeon and anesthesiologist to be aware of the diagnosis and the medications.
- **Insomnia and sleep apnea**—Weight gain is worsened by steroids, which may lead to obstructive sleep apnea (OSA). The stress and fatigue produced by OSA may then interfere with response to treatment. Diagnosing and treating OSA is very important in order to reduce fatigue in these patients.
- **Mental stress, anxiety, and depression**—Prednisone may worsen depression. Occasionally, mania is produced by steroids. Psychiatric consultation is rarely needed.
- **Physical illness**—Infections such as bronchitis, flu, common cold, and gastroenteritis are common triggers.

- **Pain**—Acute and chronic pain may lead to worsening of MG symptoms. Medications used to treat pain may lead to exacerbation.
- **Heat**—Heat (including hot showers or baths, sunbathing, saunas, hot tubs, and hot food or drink) slows down neuromuscular transmission. Dysphagia usually improves with ice cream and worsens with hot drinks.
- **Sunlight or bright lights** affect the eyes. Dark glasses are very useful to avoid glare.
- **Some medications** (a list is provided in the comments on Case #27)
- **Tonic water** (due to quinine content)
- **Low potassium levels or low thyroid levels**

> *"Dark glasses are very useful to avoid glare induced diplopia."*

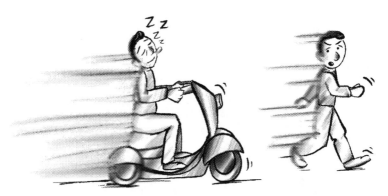

You are supposed to take a nap in the afternoon

# Case #30

## HEALTHY LIFESTYLE AND GIVE YOURSELF A BREAK

"I will take the weight gain...versus the double vision and everything else that comes with it."

My earliest symptom was a left droopy eyelid and sometimes a right droopy eyelid. I also had loss of my peripheral vision. I couldn't really move my eyes side to side, so I would have to turn my whole head to look at things. I didn't even realize my eyelid was even drooping because I couldn't feel it drooping. It wasn't until my friends noticed and asked what was wrong with my eye or if I was sleepy or something that I became aware of it.

My eye drooping was not to the point of closing, but the muscle weakness was causing my eye to droop just enough that people were noticing. Eventually, I also started to experience double vision, so to help with that I used to close one eye to help me see, especially when driving or doing anything, really. I had gone to an optometrist to see if something else was going on, because at the time I didn't know anything about myasthenia gravis. My optometrist referred me to another doctor who ran some tests and diagnosed me with myasthenia gravis. I was then finally referred to a myasthenia gravis specialist. The time from the start of the symptoms until I received a diagnosis was about one year.

When I first heard the diagnosis, I was pretty devastated, because I wasn't sure if things were going to get progressively worse or if these symptoms were permanent. This is because at the time, my symptoms were the worst they had ever been. My vision was pretty bad, and I started to get weakness in my extremities, like my arms and legs. I tried to eat better and start exercising, but my legs would give out. I couldn't carry things, because when I did, it felt like somebody was pushing down on my arms, even when I was holding something really light. I couldn't open doors, just because my muscles couldn't do it.

My muscle weakness progressed to where I was having a hard time breathing. I also started to have difficulty chewing and swallowing, so I tried to change the foods I was eating or tried not to eat as much to avoid having difficulties. So, in the beginning, I was in pretty bad shape, but luckily it got better.

The first medication I started taking was Mestinon, and that really helped improve the symptoms for about six to eight hours, until it had to be taken again. For some reason, there were a couple of side effects as well. It affected me when I was eating, causing a sort of acid reflux that was really bad, and the medication also caused some sweating as well, but that was all. I didn't have any other treatments other than the Mestinon, which really seemed to help. I also noticed that improving my diet seemed to really help.

I would stick to the doctor's plan and take the medication every day, but now I have been taking it lightly, just when I feel symptoms really. I deal with muscle fatigue by giving myself more rest at the end of things. If I used to try to exercise, I would be completely wiped out from small amounts of physical exertion, so instead I try to do something that has a longer resting period.

I notice I have the biggest relapses when I have a cold. I guess it affects my whole system So usually, if I have a cold or something, it worsens my symptoms. When this happens, the doctors just increase my dose of medication. In the beginning, I used to take the medication two or three times a day, and the doctor would scale it back down. However, when my symptoms worsened, they would start putting me on more medication to control the symptoms.

Dealing with myasthenia gravis affected me mentally. I felt like I was easily stressed because things that were sort of easy before were a lot more challenging, so I would get very frustrated. It also affected my attitude, because I would have to put in a little more effort for basic things. It affected my confidence and daily happiness, I guess. It was very frustrating.

What helped me deal with MG was improving my diet and exercising. In the beginning, I tried to exercise more, but I struggled because I would fall down at first, since my legs were not strong enough. But I kept trying, and that helped me. I am not sure, but since my diet and my whole lifestyle before was so unhealthy, maybe that's what caused my symptoms to present a little more aggressively. Making that change to my health and lifestyle seemed to help me a lot.

> *"I felt like I was easily stressed because things that were sort of easy before were a lot more challenging."*

**Expert Comment:**

The first six months after the diagnosis are probably the hardest. After that, the disease will be controlled with a small maintenance dose of medications. Also, the longer the disease, the more benign it becomes, and the lower the probability of relapse. The chance of permanent remission without medication also increases with age.

Naps are very refreshing. That is a fact. Periods of rest are frequently needed. Repetitive actions are very tiring.

A change in lifestyle is often helpful, and MG is usually a wakeup call. Weight reduction, a healthy diet, and a better sleep pattern are very helpful.

> *"The first six months after the diagnosis are probably the hardest."*

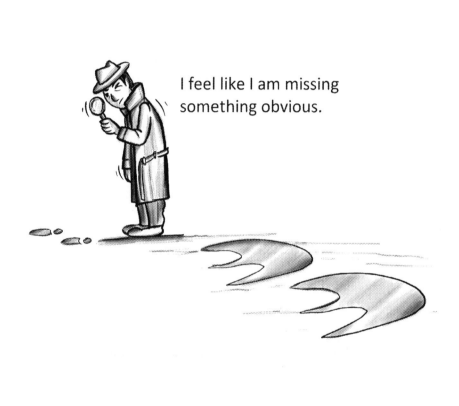

I feel like I am missing something obvious.

# Case #31

## NEVER GIVE UP AND NEVER STOP LOOKING FOR ANSWERS

"If you're familiar with prednisone, you know that after about three weeks, you want to eat everything in sight."

The earliest symptoms I experienced were double vision, blurriness, and some distorted vision. First I thought it was just my glasses; maybe I just needed to up my prescription, or maybe there was a little tilt on my lens. I was thinking it was something minor, but later I discovered that it was something much greater.

Around the time when my symptoms first began, about three years ago, I started working for an eye doctor. It was such a coincidence that my vision problems started about the same time that I started working for an eye doctor.

Before seeing the specialist, I can't even tell you the number of doctors I saw. I saw the optometrist I was working for and explained my symptoms. He referred me out to an ophthalmologist, who was his best friend. That doctor couldn't figure out what it was. He just didn't know and said he was smart enough to admit that he didn't know. That doctor then referred me out to a neuro-specialist who thought I had a tumor. He wasn't wrong: I do have a very small tumor. That is very common. Apparently, one out of three patients has it.

The doctor had some CAT scans done: two head scans and two of my rotator cuff and my eyes. The doctor thought I might have multiple sclerosis and that was what was causing my symptoms. So it had just been one thing after the other.

I went to a different hospital, and a couple of doctors there couldn't figure it out. They wanted to do cosmetic surgery on one of my eyes, because the drooping was just that bad. The symptoms would switch over from one eye to the other. But at this point, the symptoms were staying on the right eye, so they wanted to do cosmetic surgery to remove part of my eyelid on my right eye. Thank the Lord they didn't, because looking back and knowing my diagnosis, I could have had a little piece of my eye gone for no reason. It also would've been uneven, and I would have had to do the other side. I am just thankful that my MG doctor figured it out and both of my eyes are now back open.

I wasn't officially diagnosed with myasthenia gravis until I was referred to a specialist in the MG field. When the doctor first told me the diagnosis, I was scared to death. Nobody wants to have a disease that they have to deal with for the rest of their life. First you think, *Oh my God, my life is over.* Not literally, but you realize that you have to take medication for the rest of your life. It just felt like it was a hindrance.

But now that I have been living with it, it's hard to explain, but it's not as bad as it seems. As you go on and live, you think more about the quality of your life, and you think about being there for your children, and you just have to do what you have to do. It is what it is.

I feel like the best way I coped with the diagnosis and the symptoms was due to family support. I don't know if what I did was even truly coping. I don't have any family here where I live, since they live about two hours away from me. But I have my husband here. I do sometimes feel bad because when I have a relapse and my double vision comes back, my husband has to drive me everywhere. But all I can say is, my husband has played a huge part in helping me. He is always going to the doctor with me, being very patient with me, and this all takes time, because he has to drive me to work sometimes. There are times when he has to come get me when I have pulled over on the side of the road because I can't see when it's raining.

> **"I could have had a little piece of my eye gone for no reason."**

I just feel like you have to have some kind of family support or some kind of group support. I feel like I couldn't have done it alone, because it's been a lot of hard nights sometimes where I've just been upset and I've cried. It's very hard on the whole family, not just me. It takes the whole family, but it's good to know that you're not alone.

At first, the doctor put me on Mestinon, but it didn't work well with my stomach and my digestive system. It was awful. I couldn't even get off the bathroom floor one time. I had to call the ambulance. It was also causing me to pass out at work, so I'm just glad I no longer have to take it. The doctor told me I could take the Mestinon if I wanted to, but I opted out of it because it was not working for me at all.

Instead, I was put on prednisone, which is what I am on now. Although prednisone is great, it just wasn't enough to control my symptoms. I needed more medication. He did add another medication, which I have to take for two years, and right now I feel like everything's going great. I started taking it last week, and I haven't had any side effects yet. If I do have side effects, I'll let the doctor know, but for now I am pleased with the medication I am currently on.

I never tried to change the dosage of my medication, and I always followed what my doctor said. Even when my stomach was hurting and the medication sent me to the hospital, I just tried to get through it. I never tried to deviate from the plan.

Later in my treatment plan, my doctor tried to taper me off the steroids, but I am part of the 15 percent of people with MG who have a relapse in symptoms if the steroid dosage is too low. So of course, with my luck, we had to increase my steroid dosage. When I first started experiencing a relapse in symptoms, I started to panic, because I was so used to seeing one picture. Then, over the weekend, I was watching TV and realized something was wrong—that something had changed.

When you start seeing that your vision is distorted and your eyes are trying to catch up with your brain, it's all in slow-mo. I would start moving my glasses up and down because I was trying to see if it was my glasses. But you realize no, this is not your glasses. It's just a downer, and you think to yourself, *Oh my God, this can't be happening. I was doing so well for almost a year and now it's back to this.* It is so frustrating.

> **"I started to panic, because I was so used to seeing one image."**

I am on 60 milligrams now, which is fine with me, as long as my eyes are back open. Just over the weekend, my double vision came back, and my eye started closing. Thankfully, yesterday, my double vision was gone, and I'm back to normal. Tapering down the steroid dosage is the only situation that has caused me to have a relapse; other than that, nothing else has caused me to relapse.

Also, to make sure I don't take medications that worsen my condition, my doctor gave me a list of medications I can and can't take with MG. The doctor said that if another doctor puts me on some other medication, I would have to clear it with the specialist first.

The only side effect I have had from the steroids would be gaining weight. When I started, I was 120 pounds, and now I think I am 165 pounds. But you know what? I will take that. I will take the weight gain and go on a diet or whatever it takes to maintain my weight if that's what makes me happy, versus the double vision and everything else that comes with it. I don't care about gaining weight. I'll take the weight gain. Luckily, that's the only side effect I've had from the steroids.

MG has affected my ability to exercise. It's really hard to place what is causing what exactly, because I am on other medications as well. But I find that I have a lot of numbness in my hands and legs. I don't have any more of the chewing, speaking, and clumsiness I was having before I started on prednisone. But before I started taking prednisone, it was a challenge to walk up the stairs, and I was tired all the time. My legs were hurting, and it was just exhausting. I felt like it was a fight against my own body. I found that the best way to cope with the fatigue was to just do less. I could not exercise or do anything strenuous.

Before I started taking medication, the only thing that helped the double vision was to hold my head at an angle. My head needed to be tilted up in order to see one clear picture. It was aggravating, because I had to do it on the daily, especially when I had to drive. I would have my head tilted for so long that my neck would hurt so badly.

I just want to tell everyone to never give up and to never stop looking for answers. My journey started with my optometrist, who wouldn't stop. He used all his resources. He had so many other doctors he knew, he was well connected, and he got me to my current specialist. I had to go through all the crazy diagnoses to a point where they said I had bowel syndrome and even MS. They said I had it all. It was serious.

I just want to tell everybody out there to stay the course. I know it's hard, because they take you off medication, put you on medication, and take you off again. You feel like a research project. It is all trial and error. They kind of see what it is to see if they can fix it. It's a lot of money, and it's a lot of time.

However, I think from where I was to where I am today, I wouldn't take anything back, not even the insurance claims and the money that I spent on all kinds of stuff that I don't even know. But I couldn't get here if I didn't go through what I went through before. So try to have more support, and just never give up. Never take no for an answer, because we know deep down in our heart what's right for us. If you feel like this is not the answer, then don't go with it. Keep searching for the answer till you find it.

> **"I just want to tell everyone to never give up and to never stop looking for answers."**

## Expert Comment:

Eyelid surgery for ptosis is a bad idea, because ptosis will return within a few months. Most plastic surgeons ask for clearance from a neurologist before surgery. Yes, some cases of ptosis may benefit from surgery, especially those related to muscle disease, but MG must be excluded as a cause or these diseases must be confirmed.

On feeling scared to death: This is not an easy diagnosis to take. Being diagnosed with a disease that you're hearing about for the first time can be shocking. It is important that the clinician spends time to explain and answer questions. The idea behind this book is to alleviate fear and provide a better understanding of the disease and how to cope with it.

Family support is crucial, especially during the first few months after the diagnosis when side effects and the disease may force a change in lifestyle. Also, the elderly will need some help with administration of medications. Confusion may have catastrophic effects on treatment.

Never give up: This kind of encouragement is needed, especially in dealing with an unpredictable disease like MG. Giving up is usually associated with poor compliance with medications and frequent relapses and morbidity.

Recurrence of symptoms after the prednisone is lowered occurs in 15 percent of cases. In these situations, a steroid-sparing agent is usually added in order to enable a more successful tapering after a few months.

> *"The idea behind this book is to alleviate fear and provide a better understanding of the disease and how to cope with it."*

> *"Every time I would try to push through,*
> *I would start feeling worse."*

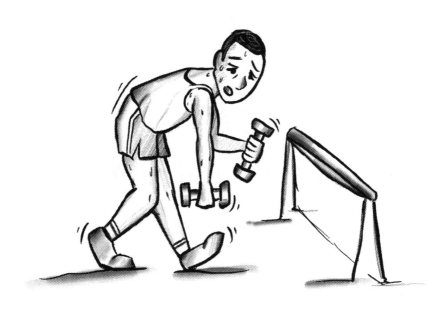

Another mile and I will rest

# Case #32

## DON'T EXERCISE TO EXHAUSTION

"Normally, when people get sick… it's a bad thing.
In my case, it was a blessing in disguise."

My earliest symptoms were an inability to swallow and shortness of breath. I was originally seeing an ENT (ear, nose, and throat) physician for throat problems and inability to swallow, and he was giving me therapy for it. I want to say I was seeing him for about a year, maybe a year and a half.

However, I had an attack during one of my appointments while I was working with a speech therapist, and she alerted the doctor that something unusual was going on. He brought me into the room and proceeded to do some tests. He then told me that he thought I had myasthenia gravis. I didn't really have any reaction to the diagnosis. I have glaucoma, and I've had skin cancer, so hearing the diagnosis, my reaction was, "Well, that's just life." He referred me to my first neurologist, who did a Tensilon test and confirmed the diagnosis.

At the time, I was in my fifties, and the neurologist wanted me to have a thymectomy. My thymectomy was scheduled for the morning but was delayed to the late afternoon, and I was having an IVIG treatment done before the surgery. I remember sitting there thinking, "I'm going to have them open up my chest, and I'm doing just fine. This strikes me as a little bit insane." I really had an urge to get up and walk out, but I didn't.

The thymectomy involves three days in the hospital and about two weeks to recover. By then, since I was only on Mestinon, my symptoms were exacerbated. They were worse than they ever were before. So, I was not particularly pleased with the surgery from that standpoint.

I called the doctor up and said, "I've got a problem."

His response was, "Well, when you're bad enough to go to the ER, that's when we'll treat you." Wonderful. I was not a fan of this doctor.

I went back to my ENT physician, and he recommended a different neurologist. I went to see this new neurologist, who said he wouldn't have done the thymectomy, because he believes that a thymectomy for people over the age of fifty just makes their symptoms worse. Anyway, he decided he would use plasmapheresis and IVIG to maintain my condition, since he was not a fan of immunosuppression.

I found this doctor to be wonderful—probably one of the best bedside manners I have ever seen. I kept going to this doctor for several years. He treated me multiple times, mostly with plasmapheresis and sometimes with IVIG whenever I had symptoms. Unfortunately, he developed cancer and took a break from his practice, and his partners did not want to treat MG. So, I was referred to a different neurologist.

I have been seeing this neurologist ever since, and he is the one who put me on immunosuppressant's and prednisone, and has since tapered me off. I think for the time that I've been here, I've had two times when my symptoms flared up. One time was due to a viral infection, which has a tendency to exacerbate symptoms. Both times I had my symptoms flare up, the doctor would run up the prednisone dose really high.

> *"If you're familiar with prednisone, you know that after about three weeks, you want to eat everything in sight."*

If you're familiar with prednisone, you know that after about three weeks, you want to eat everything in sight. I'm still trying to lose the weight, but I'm off prednisone, and I'm only on immunosuppressant's. Currently, I am backing off the suppressant, which makes me a happy camper.

When I first had the MG symptoms, the only thing I knew that would help me was to just sit quietly when I received my food and wait it out. It was very, very frustrating, because you're sitting there, you just ordered lunch, and there's a plate of food there. You take two bites, and you're done. The worst thing about it was if I had a margarita, I was toast. So, I gave up alcohol, and I haven't really gone back.

The situation was disheartening, because you're really hungry but you can't eat. Luckily, in the early mornings, I didn't have symptoms, and if I did, they were very, very seldom. The symptoms would develop by noon, and by the evening, if I was going to get the symptoms, that's when they really hit.

The first treatment I had was the thymectomy. After the procedure, I was fine for about two weeks, but the symptoms came back, and they came back worse than I had ever had before. After the thymectomy, the only medication I was given was Mestinon. Until I had the thymectomy, Mestinon didn't work, but after the thymectomy, it did. What is interesting is the Mestinon only had an impact on me if I had my symptoms under control.

For example, once I did plasmapheresis or IVIG to control my symptoms, Mestinon would actually help me—but before those treatments, it didn't help. My doctor would put me on Mestinon and I would be fine for six months, until the symptoms would rear their ugly head back in and I couldn't function. Then we would do plasmapheresis or IVIG, and I'd be good for another six months. Thankfully, I haven't taken Mestinon in years, because I haven't had attacks.

In terms of treatments, I have had no bad side effects with the IVIG treatments. The IVIG is an IV you have for several days, but it's no big deal. The plasmapheresis is just a pain in the patootie, because you're trapped. In plasmapheresis, you spend a lot of time doing the transfer, and they do it in a series of three to five sessions in a row. So, there's a good chunk of time that goes with the treatment. But I didn't have any bad side effects with the plasmapheresis.

Plasmapheresis and IVIG were helpful because their effect is almost instantaneous. You go in with symptoms, and after the first treatment, they're pretty much gone. Unlike plasmapheresis or IVIG, prednisone takes time to bring the symptoms down. The last time I took it, about three years ago, it took about two or three weeks after starting the prednisone before the symptoms relaxed. So, prednisone is not an instant cure, but I wasn't bad enough that I needed an instant cure.

I am always compliant with my doctor's plan for medication. The only time I have not been compliant was when my neurologist was planning to reduce my prednisone dosage, but when I saw him, he decided he didn't want to do it. So, I waited a month, and then I started reducing it on my own. The next time I came into the office to see him, the medication was already reduced, and he didn't say anything.

I have had the same general practitioner since the mid-1980s. When I first went in there with MG, she admitted she was not really familiar with it, so she brought out her manual and we read it together. She now has other patients who have MG, and she is very cognizant of drug reactions. There are some antibiotics that are really bad for patients with MG, and at the time, there was a limited variety of antibiotics I could have, so she said, "This is the only one I can give you." She explained the side effects, and I decided forget it—I would go without the antibiotics. So, whenever she prescribes something, we go through it together and make sure it is fine to take with my MG.

In terms of myasthenia affecting my physical activity, I try to make sure I don't exercise to exhaustion. I get regular massage and chiropractic treatments. My massage person does very deep work, and every once in a while, he will be very intense. For instance, he worked on my legs one time for an hour, and when I left there, they were completely exhausted. After the session, I was walking over an uneven surface, and I fell because my legs were really tired. So, I am cognizant of that, and I try to watch out for that, but I don't exercise to exhaustion—or if I do, I make sure to sit and take a break.

My problem with steroids was the weight gain. I gained a hundred pounds while on steroids. Since I've been off them, I'm losing weight, and I have been doing intermittent fasting to help me lose weight too. When you're on steroids, it's a real pain to try to lose weight; the weight just creeps up on you. Now I've gone in the opposite direction and have lost fifteen pounds in three months, especially since I am off the steroids.

Since one of my doctors had a displeasure with doing immunosuppressant and prednisone because of the side effects, the first immunosuppressant drug he tried was cyclosporin, and I developed kidney and bladder stones. So we went back to IVIG. When I switched to the new neurologist, I got on Imuran. This is to say, steroids work and Imuran works. I'm relatively symptom-free, so I'm not particularly concerned about the long-term effects. I know that long-term use of steroids has detrimental effects, but I am still alive. I suspect at some point, MG may shorten my life somewhat, but what can you do?

> ## "So, prednisone is not an instant cure, but I wasn't bad enough that I needed an instant cure."

**Expert Comment:**

Alcohol drinking is not particularly contraindicated in MG. However, too much drinking tends to worsen weakness and fatigue, and it may worsen the effect on the liver of some medications used to treat MG. Similarly, there is no special dietary regimen that is advised in MG patients. A low-carb diet is recommended with steroids to avoid weight gain. I advise patients with dysphagia to moisten solid foods with gravy, sauce, broth, butter, mayonnaise, sour cream, or yogurt; to choose chicken or fish instead of tougher meats; and to try crumbly food such as crackers, rice, cookies, nuts, chips, or popcorn.

IVIG and PLEX are used for myasthenic crises when breathing is compromised or in severe exacerbation when patients cannot swallow medications. The onset of action is hours to days, and the duration is weeks. They are temporizing agents. When steroids and steroid agents are ineffective or tolerated, IVIG or PLEX become chronic therapies.

Steroid-sparing agents such as azathioprine, methotrexate, mycophenolate, and cyclosporine are used when steroid tapering is associated with recurrence of symptoms. Most of them need months to work, and the steroid dose may be lowered by then.

While heavy exercises are not recommended in MG, mild exercises to improve strength, endurance, and mental health are recommended.

> ## "Alcohol drinking is not particularly contraindicated in MG."

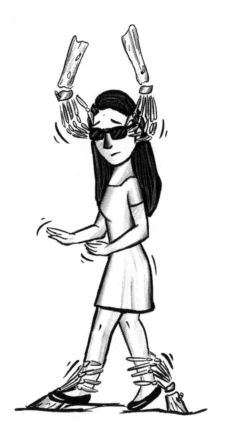

Weak legs! Blurred vision!
It must be the zombie invasion.

# Case #33

## What Was Wrong with Me?

"It feels like my mind and my body are fighting each other."

My earliest symptom was extreme fatigue. It started out where I'd be tired, and I would have to lay down and rest. If I didn't rest, I would literally feel like I was getting sick. My body wasn't giving me a choice. Normally, when you're healthy and you don't have myasthenia gravis, everybody gets tired from time to time, but you can push through it. I used to always be able to do that, but it started getting to the point where I couldn't push through. Every time I would try to push through, I would start feeling worse.

I started getting really depressed, because I have a lot of kids and grandkids, and we are always on the run, doing stuff with everybody. There would be times when we would have fun things planned with the kids, and because I was having a bad day and was feeling extremely fatigued, I couldn't go. I would have to just lay down and rest. It'd be one of the kids' baseball games or dancing with the girls, just anything fun like that, and I couldn't go. This made me so sad, because I didn't know what was wrong with me.

I was going to my OB/GYN for a regular checkup, and I told her what was going on. She did a lot of testing on me, including blood work and checking my hormones. I was low on a few hormones, and she wanted to start me on BioTE—a hormone replacement therapy in the form of a pill. However, something just kept telling me, *Don't do it.*

I am not sure if it was instinct, but I didn't end up doing it because I didn't like the idea of taking a pill that might have side effects I couldn't control. If I started feeling sick or felt like I was having bad side effects, I couldn't just stop taking it. It's in your body at that point, so I didn't feel right about doing it.

I didn't do the BioTE therapy, but I did start on a hormone cream that I would just rub on myself once a day. The cream was helping a little bit, but not like it was supposed to. I went several years not knowing what was wrong with me.

In 2017, I started noticing that my eyesight was doing something weird. I called it tunnel vision. Now I know they call it *double vision* or *diplopia*. At the time, I didn't know what it was, but it was really hard to focus sometimes. I was not seeing things clearly.

It's really confusing when you're trying to walk and you can't see things clearly. It's hard to explain. But I didn't like to walk around because of it. After I noticed the odd vision, I ended up getting sick with the flu in December of 2017. I went to see a doctor, and he started me on Tamiflu. At this point, I was having really weird vision problems, and I could not get up or see straight. It's almost like I was drunk.

I thought it was a side effect of the medicine, so I kept telling my family that I was never taking this medication again. I told them that the medication had messed me up so badly that I couldn't stand or see.

They said, "But you were having that problem before you got sick."

I said, "Yeah, but not this bad. Now it has gotten worse."

Even when I told my doctor about it, the doctor just looked at me funny and said, "That is not one of the side effects of the medication."

I replied, "Well, it did to me."

> **"This made me so sad, because I didn't know what was wrong with me."**

Right after I got over the flu, my left eye started getting really small and started to droop. I thought I was having a stroke. I also started having trouble with my voice. It felt like my vocal cords were strained, because my voice sounded really weird. I noticed when I would stop talking for a minute and rest my vocal cords, then the next time I would talk, my voice would sound normal for a little bit, and then it would get weird again within just a few minutes.

I was worried, so I went to my family doctor and asked her, "What is my eye doing? What is wrong with me? Am I having a stroke? What's going on?"

It just so happens that my doctor knew a little bit about MG and its symptoms. She said, "Okay, it could be one of two things. So, I'm going to test you for both." She thought it was Bell's palsy, possibly, but then she stated that if it was Bell's palsy, it would cause one side of my face to droop, not just my eyes. She said, "It might be something else, so I'm going to do some blood work."

She did blood work, which took a few days. We got the results back, and that's when we knew for sure that it was MG. I am grateful she knew enough about the symptoms of MG to test for it, or else I wouldn't know what was going on with me.

Normally, when people get sick, for example with the flu, it's a bad thing. In my case, it was a blessing in disguise. I had been going through extreme fatigue for years, and I knew something was wrong with me, but we just couldn't figure it out. When I got sick with the flu, it caused my MG symptoms to flare up enough that my doctor was able to diagnose me within that week. I am so grateful she diagnosed me, because I went at least three years without knowing what was going on.

When I first heard the diagnosis, it was upsetting, because my whole life I've always been a very healthy person. I love to be active to keep in shape, whether by working out, playing with my kids, or running the heavy laundry up the stairs. I've always had the energy to do that. However, with MG, I would work out until I started having that fatigue. Then I didn't have the energy to do it anymore.

After learning all the information about MG, I knew that my life was never going to be the same. However, I am thankful that my doctor said it is not a terminal illness. It's just something that you have to adjust your life to, because your body is not what it used to be.

> **"Why me, I've always been a very healthy person."**

At first I feared what I was facing, because I didn't know anything about it, and neither did my doctors. I started to search online, but my doctor warned me that a lot of the things online are not accurate. I was advised not to look online and instead trust the information that the doctor was giving me. I don't know if it's a learning process at this point, but adjusting to the disease is something I have to deal with on a daily basis.

Right after my family doctor diagnosed me with MG, she sent me to a physical therapist and a neurologist. At first, I didn't know why I needed a physical therapist, but it was to learn some new exercises with my face to open my eyes more. When I went to see the neurologist, he started me on Mestinon.

The medicine helped my eye open a little bit. It didn't look all the way normal, but it was better than it had been. As for my voice, the Mestinon helped it a little bit, but not very much. The main problem with Mestinon is that it only lasts for a few hours, and you have to take it again every four to six hours. I didn't like the medicine, and at the same time, I was still having that weird vision. So it didn't really help. But I wasn't as confused or as disoriented.

I remember, before the medications, there were several times when I tried to go to the grocery store but couldn't. My vision was so bad that I was focusing on just trying to walk straight, because I didn't want people thinking that I was drunk or on drugs. It was so difficult. Something so easy that we take for granted like going to the store, I couldn't do. Walking to the bathroom or walking to get something to eat in the kitchen—I couldn't do it. It was just so irritating, because I couldn't see straight.

After I saw that neurologist, he didn't know much about myasthenia gravis, so he referred me to another neurologist who was an expert in the field. He asked if I would be willing to travel to the city to see him. At that point, I was willing to do anything. I said, "Yes, we know what I have, now I want to learn how to deal with it. I don't want to be like this for the rest of my life. I have too many kids and grandkids, so I want to be as normal as I possibly can be."

I went to see the specialist, and he was very informative. He placed me on a high dose of prednisone, 50 mg every day, and that really helped me. The prednisone started helping me with my eye, which started to look more normal. It's still a little bit smaller than my right eye, but it's not as noticeable as it was. The prednisone also helped my voice sound back to normal. I've been talking a lot, and it's not changing, so I am thankful for that medicine.

My neurologist was able to wean me down gradually. I went from taking 50 milligrams every day to 15 milligrams every other day. Some days, I feel pretty good, while other days, I don't feel 100 percent normal, energy-level wise. When I do feel good, I can do a whole lot that day. But there are other days when I can only do a little bit, and then I have to sit down to rest. The day will consist of me working, then resting.

That's another thing I hate. I feel like my body is dependent on this medicine, and I hate that. I'm glad this medicine is helping me, and I know once I take it, I'm going to feel better, but I hate that I need that medicine to feel better.

Once I started taking the prednisone, it helped, but it also gave me strange side effects. Before taking prednisone, I was really thin. I am five feet three inches tall, and I weighed 114 pounds. I had always been very petite. The doctor told me that I was going to gain weight as a side effect of the prednisone. I was doubtful that this would apply to me, but unfortunately, I was wrong. I gained weight; I was really puffy, and I had that big moon face. I went from 114 pounds all the way up to 140 pounds. For some people, that's not a lot, but to me it is. I've only weighed that much when I was nine months pregnant with my big babies.

The medicine does have a bittersweet taste, and when I take it, the effects do make me feel better, but it also makes my muscles feel weird— not tingly or weak, just a strange feeling while I'm walking or while I'm using my arms. Although my body feels weird on the medication, I can still function. I told my doctor about the feeling it was giving me, because I wasn't sure if it was the MG or if it was a medicine. The doctor said, "The medicine is what's making your body feel like that. It's the prednisone."

Before the medicine, there was nothing that really helped me with the fatigue. My left eye was so small, and it wouldn't open as big as my right eye. So I got in the habit of holding my head back like you would when you are looking up in the sky. I did this so my eyes were on the same level, and I kept it up for a little while, but then it started making my neck hurt. My doctor mentioned it wasn't good to do it anyway, because it can cause other problems with my neck.

> ### "I feel like my body is dependent on this medicine, and I hate that."

Before I knew I had MG, I'd get so tired that I would have to go lie down and rest. Even if I just sat down for a little bit, I would automatically doze off. Then I was good to go and could do what I needed to do. Giving myself a nap is how I dealt with the fatigue. Once I was diagnosed with MG, I learned how it affects your body and that your muscles have to rest. With rest, your muscles get their strength back. However, it is aggravating when you've got a lot of stuff to do and you don't want to rest. You want to get it done, but you are too tired to push through.

I never tried to change my medication plan given to me by my doctor, because my doctor reassured me that, "I know how to treat what you have. I have a lot of patients with this, and I know what I'm doing. When I tell you to take medicine, take it the way I tell you to." He told me that there were patients of his who had tried to change the medicine because they were thinking, *Oh, I'm feeling better. I don't need this much medicine anymore.* So they'd either cut their medication themselves or they'd wean themselves off abruptly. Then they'd start having major problems like breathing problems, and they'd end up in the hospital and on a ventilator.

I stick to the doctor's plan because I know that the effects of MG on my extremities is the least of the problems, since MG can affect even more vital organs, like my heart and my lungs. I don't want to be one of those people who end up in the hospital because I didn't listen and take my medicine the way I was supposed to. There have been a couple of times when I've messed up on accident, but never on purpose.

I especially remember messing up when I had to start taking the medication every other day. I would get confused and think, *Is today my medicine day, or was it yesterday?* That's another side effect of the prednisone: it causes memory loss or confusion. What I started doing early on to prevent this was that every day I would write it down, even when I was taking the medication every other day. The paper would remind me if I took it yesterday or if I didn't take it yesterday, so I knew which day was my medicine day. Sometimes my body will naturally remind me to take it—like today, I've been feeling really tired, and I realize that I have not taken it. But I always keep track of it on paper as a reminder.

After some time, my MG specialist recommended a thymectomy. He said it would be easier to control the disease without the thymus, and the surgery could help slow the disease progression. The results from other people who have had a thymectomy before have shown little to no progression in their disease. My doctor informed me that the disease and whatever symptoms I had developed up until the time of the surgery would still be there. I was always going to have those symptoms, but we could control them, because they were not going to get worse. I was not going to develop any additional symptoms.

> **"I don't want to be one of those people who end up in the hospital because I didn't listen."**

I was interested at this point. We talked about different ways to do the surgery. I had looked it up and saw that there were two different ways to do it. One way was a sternotomy, where they cut through the breastbone; I wasn't excited about that one, since it seemed too invasive for something that was not even 100 percent guaranteed to help me. A long time ago, that was the only way they could do it. However, now they had minimally invasive surgery and robotic surgery.

My MG doctor referred me to a cardiovascular surgeon who could do a thymectomy. Unfortunately, when we went to go talk to the doctor, we found out that he only performed the surgery by doing a sternotomy. I decided the only way I was going to do the surgery was if it was done through a thoracoscopic procedure.

Thankfully, I was referred to a different doctor who performed the surgery robotically. I went to see this new surgeon, and he was very thorough. He said he could do the procedure by making only four small incisions. I even questioned him to make sure it was just as accurate and successful as the sternotomy. He reassured me that he could do everything that the sternotomy technique could do without being so invasive, because everything was magnified in the surgery.

I trusted what I was told, and on June 11, 2019, I had a thoracoscopic thymectomy. After the surgery, I was in the ICU, but I didn't have to stay on the ventilator. I guess the only bad experience I had from that whole thing was the chest tube. That was horrible, but you must have a chest tube in with all surgery. That was the most painful part of it all, honestly. Other than being really sore, I didn't have any side effects with the thymectomy.

I went home the very next day. I recovered really fast, because the robotic way is less invasive, so it's easier to heal from. The doctor told me that if I had a sternotomy, it would take about six weeks to recover. Overall, the benefits I was told about the thymectomy have been true. However, I just had it eight months ago, so it's maybe too soon to tell.

Occasionally if I'm stressed out, it can cause me to have a relapse. I have a lot of kids in the family, so there's always something to deal with. When the kids are acting out or being emotional, I've noticed it will kind of trigger my MG a little bit. I still get extreme fatigue—that's still my number-one symptom. However, if tiredness is the worst symptom I'm going to have, then I will take it. I know there are people who are going through a lot more pain than I am, so I'm not going to complain about being tired, since that's one of the easier symptoms.

It is aggravating, and I do complain when I have a lot of things to do but my body is too tired. Then I catch myself and go, "You know what? Don't complain. You're not in pain. If you just rest for a little bit, you're going to feel a lot better. You can then jump up and do some more stuff."

Going through this disease has affected me psychologically and has caused me to be really sad at times. But I got through because as a Christian, I just prayed for God to help me through it. I also knew that being sad was part of a normal grieving process because I'm adjusting to something so different from anything I've ever had to deal with.

I used to be my normal energetic self and just do everything all day long. I was constantly busy. Now, my body is making me stop and rest while my mind is still going ninety miles an hour. It feels like my mind and my body are fighting each other. This was very difficult for me, because I was raised by my father, who was an officer in the military, and he raised me to be so strong. That life is tough. When things get hard, you fight harder. You don't give up. I've always been a really strong person. So being diagnosed with MG affected me, because I knew that it was going to change me. I knew that I was not going to have the same kind of life that I used to have before I developed the MG, being strong and energetic, working out all this kind of stuff.

I made sure to raise my kids strong too. Two of them are in the military, one is in the Marines and the other is in the Navy. It can be difficult, because they know me as this strong woman, and they keep pushing me. They don't understand that I can't with the MG. I understand where their mindset is coming from, because pain is weakness leaving the body. That's what they believe. The more pain you push through, the stronger you will be. That's how I was raised, but then you see it doesn't work like that.

Some advice I would offer is to follow your doctor's advice. Whatever the doctor tells you to do, follow it exactly, because the doctor knows how to deal with this. I feel like if you have a good doctor who knows this disease very well and knows how to treat it, if you listen and do everything the doctor tells you to do, then you shouldn't have any problems.

Everybody's different; the disease affects everybody's body in different ways. Just listen to your body, the way it feels, and rest when your body tells you to rest. Don't push yourself too hard, because that can make your symptoms worse.

I trust that God's helping me through this too. He gives me what I need, when I need it. I also think it's very important to have a support group. I got into a support group in my area, but people stopped going because a hurricane hit and destroyed a lot of houses. So, we were referred to a larger support group in the city. They have guest speakers, like doctors who will come all the time to talk about MG. However, with all my kids and grandkids, it has been difficult to make the commute, especially because the meetings take place on the weekends. I haven't gone to a group meeting since, but I would love to go again and meet other people with the disease.

It especially would've been good to have had someone to talk to about my surgery. Before I had the surgery, I was really nervous about it. I really wanted to talk to somebody who'd already had the surgery so I could've had an idea of what to expect. So, if you can, I would recommend joining a support group where you can talk to people who know what you are going through or have maybe been going through it longer than you have. It would have helped me to deal with the situation a lot better and not feel so alone.

> **"I trust that God's helping me through this too. He gives me what I need, when I need it."**

**Expert Comment:**

The thymus gland is a small gland located behind the upper part of the sternum and in front of the heart level. It measures about five by three centimeters and weighs fifty grams at puberty. It is larger during childhood and shrinks during adulthood. At age seventy, it becomes a small tag that is difficult to localize unless it has a tumor.

The gland consists of lymphoid tissue, and it is part of the immune system. It helps the immune system tolerate the native tissue, and if something goes wrong with it, the immune system may start attacking the native tissue, such as the junction between the muscle and nerve, as happens in MG. Among patients with MG, 10 percent have a tumor of the thymus gland (thymoma); it is usually benign but sometimes malignant and invasive.

Removal of the thymus (thymectomy) improves the long-term remission rate of MG, especially at age twenty to forty-five years with seropositive MG and a disease duration of less than five years. These patients will have fewer relapses and need fewer admissions to the hospital and fewer medications to control the diseases. Thymectomy is indicated for all MG patients between ages eighteen and seventy years if their general condition allows.

Transsternal thymectomy is done through a sternal incision, and it takes patients longer to recover after surgery. Minimally invasive video-assisted thoracoscopic thymectomy (VAD) is less traumatic and requires less hospitalization. It is done through one or more holes in the left or right side of the chest or abdomen. This procedure has become more and more common despite the lack of controlled trials to prove its effectiveness compared to the regular sternal thymectomy. There is a concern that VAT may not excite all the thymus tissue that may infiltrate the surrounding fat. However, this risk is theoretical.

Education of patients about MG is very important and can be lifesaving. Patients need to be aware of the symptoms of relapse and how to differentiate those from side effects of medications or anxiety. They need to learn about the harmful medications, effect of diet, exercise, lifestyle changes, drug interaction, and how to cope with the disease. There are several support groups and organizations such as www.myasthenia.org (Myasthenia Gravis Foundation of America) and myaware.org (a British group to fight MG together). These websites provide information, connect people with MG, lead them to helpful resources, and update them about disease management. Also, these groups provide names of MG experts.

The issue of vaccination in MG always comes up. Flu vaccination is not contraindicated. Nasal flu vaccine consists of a live virus and is to be avoided. Pneumonia, poliomyelitis, and hepatitis B vaccinations are not contraindicated. Shingles vaccine consists of live attenuated (weakened) virus, and the risk of contracting the disease from the vaccination should be discussed with the physician.

> *"Removal of the thymus (thymectomy) improves the long-term remission rate of MG."*

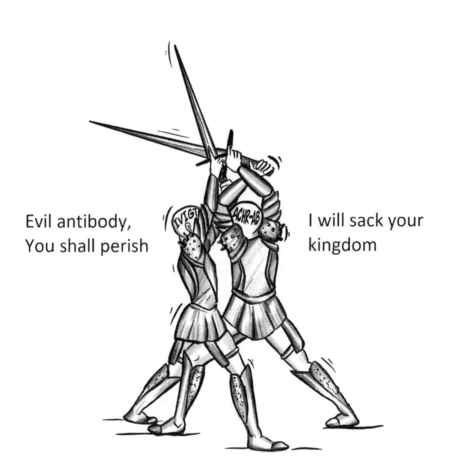

# Case #34

## THE IVIG WORKED FOR THREE MONTHS

"I believe that we become what we think, and
I think I am more than my diagnoses."

My first symptoms started about ten or twelve years ago. My left eye was going down, so I went to see an optometrist, since I thought it was an eye problem or something. The optometrist couldn't do anything, so she had me go see a neurologist.

The neurologist ordered some tests for me, and finally he said I had myasthenia gravis. From the start of symptoms, it took about two to three months to finally get a diagnosis. Once I was diagnosed, the doctor gave me a half a pill of pyridostigmine. I don't remember how many milligrams he gave me, but it didn't work. I didn't have any bad side effects, it just didn't work.

I went back to him, and he said, "Well, take the whole pill." That didn't work either. So I left, for a long time—a couple of years so—and went to find another neurologist in a different city. When I found a new neurologist, I was told to take the pyridostigmine three times a day and long-acting Mestinon 180 mg tablets twice a day.

The medication made me feel better the next morning, but after I started going to work, my eyes went down again. It helped a little bit for a couple of months, and then my symptoms were back, because my throat was getting too tight, and I couldn't swallow. So it didn't help me. Also, the

180 milligram pills were very expensive. I took that medication for a couple of years, and I was wasting a lot of money. So I decided to change doctors.

The new doctor checked me into the hospital because I was having an MG crisis. That's what he told me: "You are having a crisis." I was having symptoms in my throat, I couldn't swallow, and my eyes were drooping a lot. He put me in the hospital for an IVIG that cost $10,000 each shot. The hospital bill was $150,000 for four days. Staying in the hospital for four days didn't help much. The IVIG worked for three months, but then later on, the symptoms came back. I noticed it stopped working because I used to be able to whistle really loud, and after the IVIG stopped working, I couldn't. That's the only way I knew it was affecting me in my mouth, my throat, and my eyelids.

So I went to see an MG specialist, and he helped me a lot. The doctor exchanged the pills I was taking for methotrexate, eight pills every week. This medication helped a lot; I felt very good. He told me, "If you feel better in a couple of years, you can go have a surgery to take the thymus out." He referred me another doctor to perform the surgery, and that doctor did an operation about a month ago, and I feel great now.

The only stress I had with the thymectomy was that I couldn't drive, because sometimes I would see double. That was the only thing that I was worried about, but everything turned out fine. After the surgery, I haven't experienced any relapses in symptoms. I didn't have any side effects with the surgery.

My MG doctor told me to keep the prednisone for another year. I don't know why I am still taking the steroids, because I feel good, but he told me I had to take 10 mg of the prednisone for another year. Since I had to keep taking the steroids, the doctor said I needed to take some calcium and Vitamin D.

> **"The IVIG worked for three months, but then later on, the symptoms came back."**

I am currently retired, but when I first started experiencing MG symptoms, I was working. I worked in construction, and whenever my eyes went down, I was seeing double. When I was driving, I was seeing double. Nothing helped ease the symptoms until I was given a whole bunch of medication from the doctor, which helped a little bit, but then my eyes were drooping again.

When I was first diagnosed with MG, I didn't know what it was. The doctor told me it was myasthenia gravis, and I was thinking, *What the heck is that?*

My daughter goes with me to every doctor's appointment. I was glad she was with me, because I remember one of the doctors scared the heck out of me. The doctor said, "If you don't take the medicine that I'm giving you, you're going to die." It was said just like that. She told me that she had a case where a lady died because she didn't take the medication. After hearing that, I decided I wanted to go see another doctor. I changed doctors, and the next doctor was the one who said I was in crisis and sent me to the hospital.

Luckily, MG didn't affect my ability to exercise, because I do some exercise every night. So my activity wasn't affected. I asked one of my doctors, "Can I do exercise? Can I still work?"

He said, "Yeah, you can work or exercise, whatever you want to do." So I kept doing it.

MG only really affected my vision. When it came to swallowing difficulties, I didn't know how to deal with it. I mostly had trouble when I was eating. One of the doctors sent me to the hospital to do some radiography on my throat, and they said I was doing good. I didn't have trouble with liquids, but swallowing food gave me a little bit of trouble.

The double vision was difficult to deal with. If I had to go see the doctor, my daughter always came with me so she could drive. That's the only way I could do it. Especially if I had to drive to the city, that's a lot of traffic, so I couldn't do it.

One of the main stressors I had with MG was not being able to drive. Back when I did construction, I had to drive back and forth to work. It was a lot. So, it was very stressful having to drive with my vision troubles. These vision troubles also made it difficult for me to do my construction job. Every time I went a little higher, I would see double. I couldn't do my job. That is the only stress I had; other than that, it wasn't too bad.

The main side effect I have with the steroids is they get my sugar levels way high. That's why I have to go exercise every night. Even though I'm retired, I'm still moving around to exercise.

Some last things I want to mention is I believe exercising helps. I saw on the internet one time, a long time ago, that if I lift heavy things or do some running, it's going to help me, but I'm too old for that. I didn't do it, anyway.

MG hasn't affected me really badly. The only thing was that my family was worried because I couldn't drive. I had to go to work at that time, so they worried about it too much.

> **"One of the main stressors I had with MG was not being able to drive."**

**Expert Comment:**

Prednisone is the mainstay of treatment of MG. It addresses the actual pathological process by suppressing the immune attack against the muscle part of the nerve–muscle junction. The average maintenance dose is 10–20 mg every other day. The duration of treatment is not established, and every two to four years, an attempt is made to lower the amount further if no relapse occurs. About a quarter of all patients may be able to live without it eventually, especially those who had a thymectomy. On the other hand, IVIG and PLEX work for several weeks only.

> **"About a quarter of all patients may be able to live without prednisone eventually, especially those who had a thymectomy."**

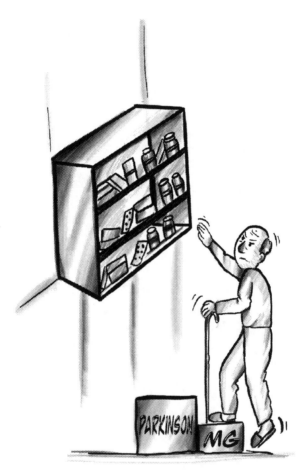

Obstacles are stepping stones

# Case #35

## I Think I Am More than My Diagnoses

My first symptoms of myasthenia gravis were a drooping of my left eyelid and double vision. I was diagnosed with Parkinson's disease in 2012 and saw a few different doctors to manage it. I do not remember who it was, but someone recommended that I schedule an appointment with an oculoplastic surgeon to have my eyelid evaluated. The surgeon performed an eyelift on my eye, hoping that would clear up the double vision. Unfortunately, the double vision remained after my eye surgery.

The oculoplastic surgeon then referred me to a neuro-ophthalmologist in Texas. Upon evaluating my vision, the ophthalmologist made an emergency referral to a different doctor in another state. My new doctor stayed in the office after hours in order to evaluate me and in turn sent me to the emergency room for further evaluation. Honestly, I am still not sure what that doctor suspected, but I was given a clean bill of health regarding that scare. Two months after my initial symptoms, my doctor diagnosed me with MG.

The diagnosis was something that I had never heard of, so I researched it online. When I understood it, I took it on as just another issue to deal with and accommodate. My father had Parkinson's disease, as did several of his siblings, so I had always anticipated having it. When I was finally diagnosed, it was almost a non-issue, and I felt the same way about my MG diagnosis. Knowledge is power, and at that point, I knew what to expect and how to minimize the effects.

My doctor placed me on a high dose of prednisone, which had no adverse side effects on me, other than an increased appetite and subsequent weight gain. Almost three years from my diagnosis, I am now taking 5 mg of prednisone and hope to be completely weaned off of it within a year. In addition to the prednisone-induced weight gain, I am also experiencing generalized fatigue and weakness. I have very little strength and get short of breath easily. Just walking to the mailbox to get the mail can leave me out of breath.

On the days that I go grocery shopping, I come home and have to rest immediately, leaving the nonperishable groceries on the kitchen counter to be put away later. On the days that I get especially worn out, I have no energy and rest in my recliner with my dog. We both spend the day sleeping.

As I said, knowledge is power. I rely on the knowledge of my doctors when it comes to my medication. I am steadfast with my medication regimen and seek expert advice when a new medication is prescribed from any one of my physicians. That goes for over-the-counter supplements like melatonin as well. I keep multiple copies of a list of all of my medications, supplements, and dosages with me at all times and provide an updated list to my physicians. For the most part, they have already considered all of my medications, but I always want to be sure. I also verify medication interaction with my pharmacist. I guess I would rather manage my health than have my health manage me.

I consider myself to be one of the fortunate ones with both of my diagnoses: myasthenia gravis and Parkinson's disease. Both are advancing at a slow pace, and I am still independent and able to spend time with my family and friends. I believe that we become what we think, and I think I am more than my diagnoses.

> *"Knowledge is power."*

## Expert Comment:

Taking an active role in the management of the disease in collaboration with the physician and not deviating from medical advice are very important for the treatment of MG. Some patients, unfortunately, take over their management and change dosage on their own, while others are so passive they do not attempt to change their lifestyle to cope with the disease. Fatigue is common, and frequent naps are refreshing. Learning about the disease and joining support groups helps with the management. Surgery to correct a droopy eyelid is not recommended in MG, as a return of the ptosis is almost always the case.

> *"Some patients, unfortunately, take over their management and change dosage on their own."*

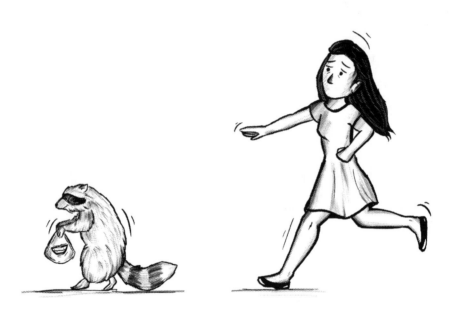

Give it back, you thief.

# Case #36

## I Lost My Nice Smile

*"I developed the moon face that is often
a part of steroid treatment."*

In the spring of 2002, I was a normal ten-year-old girl in the fifth grade. I got the flu like most of my classmates, but I also developed pneumonia. As I recovered, the fatigue from the flu never went away. It took a while to realize that there was something that definitely changed in me.

As my parents were going through a divorce, some family members thought that it was just me reacting to that. I was unable to get out of bed in the mornings without help. I could not use my tongue to move food in my mouth, so I was having to use my finger. I choked at school while eating and had to perform the Heimlich on myself. My speech became impaired; it sounded as if I was talking through my nose.

I was unable to keep up with kids my age. Longer walks became harder. I couldn't swim for long without giving up, and was unable to pull myself out of the pool. I couldn't hold myself up on a tube being pulled behind a boat that summer, and that was also the first time I experienced double vision. Looking back at pictures, my eyelids were so droopy, and I looked like I was tired all of the time.

I participated in beauty pageants, and I was unable to smile, which led to me not even placing for the first time in my life. I was a kid and had no idea what was going on with me. I just assumed that maybe I wasn't as strong as the other kids.

There were so many obvious signs as to what was going on with me, but with myasthenia gravis being so rare, it was very easily missed by my family and even medical professionals.

The most noticeable symptom, and what I started getting picked on about, was the way I talked. Several of my mom's friends said it sounded as if I needed to get my adenoids taken out. We were referred to an ENT, where we found out everything was fine with my adenoids. The ENT then suspected that I might have a cleft palate, so a barium swallow was ordered. That result came back normal. Perplexed as to what was causing me to have difficulty speaking, the doctor ordered an MRI. The MRI came back that I had a cyst on my brain, so I was referred to a neurologist.

The cyst has nothing to do with my MG and has had no effect on me whatsoever, but that cyst sent me to the right specialist, and that was my saving grace. As soon as the doctor walked in, there were no questions asked other than to my Mom: "Are her eyes always drooped like this?" It definitely threw my mom off a bit, and you could see the gears working in her head as she thought, and she said, "You know what, yes. They have been lately."

He then began doing tests that I had no idea would end up becoming my new normal when visiting the neurologist—checking my reflexes, my muscle strength, my vision and strength of eyes. It was clear that I was very weak, as I failed all of them. The doctor explained to us what myasthenia gravis was and that he expected that was what I had. It all made sense. He then referred me to a pediatric neurologist to review my case.

The pediatric neurologist was just as sure that I had myasthenia gravis. But at the words "being admitted to the hospital," the child in me broke down. I ran out of the doctor's office crying because I didn't really understand what was happening to me. After calming me down, the doctor explained that it was only for tests and to make me feel better.

> **"I participated in beauty pageants, and I was unable to smile."**

When I was finally admitted to the hospital, I was given the Tensilon test. My mom's friend was in the room. She had only known me for about six months, so the only girl she knew was the one with no smile and tired eyes. As soon as they injected the medicine into my IV, she saw me smile for the first time ever, and the light was back in my eyes. We had figured out what had made me go from a little girl full of energy to someone whose energy and strength resembled an eighty-year-old woman's. It was now October 2002, and after nearly six months of no treatment and wondering what was wrong, it was such a relief to have answers.

After a few days in the hospital and consultations with doctors, I was sent home with a prescription for Mestinon, 60 mg, three times a day. It did wonders for me, and I had a sense of normalcy back. The only side effect I seemed to have from the Mestinon was diarrhea. But the Mestinon would wear off, and my symptoms were still often there. I had reached middle school and was unable to try out for the cheerleading team due to this, which devastated me.

I was missing a lot of school because I would get too weak throughout the day. My mom was unable to keep a daytime job due to always having to leave and come get me from school. I ended up being homeschooled.

My thymus gland was enlarged slightly, but there was no thymoma. My neurologist suggested having my thymus gland removed to help ease my symptoms. She found a surgeon a few hours away who could do a minimally invasive surgery, so I did not have to go through an open heart surgery. My thymectomy was in March of 2003. The recovery was a little hard on my lungs, because the doctor went through my left lung to remove the thymus gland, and I was in the hospital for nearly a week recovering.

After I had recovered from the surgery, we noticed that my symptoms were much less severe. I also moved to taking Mestinon 180 mg timespan, which seemed to work much better. I was almost ready to have a normal middle-school life back. But that was when we realized that I had very severe scoliosis, which had been put on the back burner because of my MG diagnosis. As I was growing and also having extremely weak muscles, it seemed as if in a matter of a year, my spine went haywire. In March 2004, I had a spinal fusion to fix this.

Spending most of my middle-school years sick, in the hospital, or having surgeries really did have an effect on me. I was unable to keep up with hobbies, such as cheering. I was picked on a lot at school for the way I talked, my eyes, and my severely crooked back. But eighth grade was approaching, and I was ready to go back to school. My symptoms were much better. I was able to take my one pill in the morning and have a normal day.

Through the years, I did have times when my symptoms worsened or affected me. When I am stressed out, on my menstrual cycle, or have too much physical activity, I am much more fatigued, have trouble focusing my vision, have brain fog, have droopy eyelids, and sometimes have trouble swallowing. I am unable to exercise for more than thirty minutes without becoming very fatigued. There are instances, such as going on hikes, when I am unable to keep up with my peers.

But I have been very lucky to live a somewhat normal life with MG. I have moved a lot through my adult life, but I am always going to a neurologist at least every six months. Any doctor I have been to always gives me a list to keep on me of what medicines to avoid.

I am now twenty-eight, newly married, and the general manager of a restaurant. I work long days and am constantly on the move, but I am able to recognize when I am pushing my body too far. Rest is the best remedy for me personally and my MG.

> **"Rest is the best remedy for me personally and my MG."**

**Expert Comment:**

Myasthenia gravis in children can be devastating to their well-being and functionality. However, with proper treatment, it can be compatible with normal life. Nasal speech and loss of smile due to facial weakness are common. Children may withdraw and get depressed. Children find it hard to quit strenuous activity and hard to follow medications religiously. Side effects of prednisone are very unliked by children and teenagers, especially acne and weight gain.

Chemotherapy is to be avoided at childbearing age because it may affect fertility and pregnancy. Thymectomy is to be avoided in children, because the thymus gland has an important immunological function.

> *"Chemotherapy is to be avoided at childbearing age because it may affect fertility and pregnancy."*

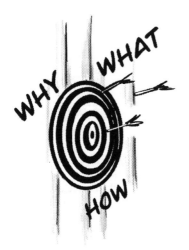
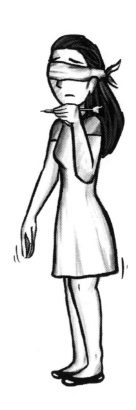

# Case #37

## HOW COULD THIS HAPPEN TO ME?

The earliest symptom I experienced with myasthenia gravis was difficulty swallowing. I would choke on certain foods, causing me to throw up. Oddly, rice seemed to be the worst food to cause difficulty swallowing. I became selective in the foods I ate and needed to eat slowly. This was followed a couple of weeks later by slurring of speech and difficulty talking for any length of time. I made an effort to limit the amount of talking I did, as I felt that my voice was failing because I was talking for too long a period of time.

Although I did not recognize it, at the same time others noticed my eyelids were drooping. I experienced some mild diplopia but did not associate that with the other symptoms. I made an appointment with my primary-care physician to determine the cause of these problems. He was not able to ascertain any physical problems that would cause these difficulties. He referred me to an ENT.

It took two to three weeks to get an appointment, during which time the symptoms became worse. The ENT could not find anything physical that would be causing the problems and referred me to a neurologist. The neurologist took a medical history and a history of the symptoms and did a physical examination. He preliminarily diagnosed me with myasthenia gravis. He ordered blood tests to confirm the diagnosis and prescribed Mestinon. He indicated that if the medication was effective, then that was a good verification of the diagnosis.

I recorded in my journal the following day: "The medicine that the doctor prescribed really worked fast. All of my symptoms went away almost immediately." With the results from the blood test being positive for MG and the success of the medication, the neurologist was able to make a final determination that I had myasthenia gravis. He referred me to see my current doctor.

The period of time from the first symptoms to the diagnosis was in excess of three months. Although I was relieved to find out the cause of my problems, my reaction to the diagnosis was perhaps one of confusion. First, I had never heard of the disease, and second, I was in great physical condition. I worked out at the gym daily, jogged regularly, rode a bicycle frequently, participated in triathlons, and ran a couple of marathons. How could this happen to me? But I was determined to beat this. I studied all I could find on the subject and tried to make the best decisions on following whatever treatment I was given.

The Mestinon was effective, but I was informed that it could not be a long-term solution. Additionally, it caused me to have diarrhea and sometimes nausea. I met with my current doctor and began my road to recovery. I began a treatment of high doses of prednisone with a period of tapering down on the dosage level. The symptoms went away quickly, and I did not need to take Mestinon at any later point.

The side effect of the prednisone was weight gain. I was always hungry and lacked energy to continue my exercise routine. I developed the moon face that is often a part of steroid treatment. The treatment went so well that I felt I really didn't need to continue the medication. Unfortunately, I had a relapse and had to start over with a high dosage of prednisone followed by tapering off.

I had an additional problem with my MG returning due to receiving the wrong anesthesia during surgery. I tried to be very careful in following the list of medications that would exacerbate the MG. I gave this to all of the physicians who treated me for other medical problems. I gave the surgeon the list and informed him that I had MG. Unfortunately, he decided to use what he always used and figured he would deal with any problems. The problem was a severe MG crisis that caused me to nearly not come out from under anesthesia. I again had to go through the high dosage of prednisone followed by tapering off. I recovered from this episode and did not experience any further problems.

> *"Always inform your surgeon that you have MG
> so that they will avoid certain medications."*

Even with the MG under control, I was still not satisfied. I did not want to always have the prospect of another reoccurrence of symptoms followed by the prednisone treatment. When the opportunity to have a thymectomy was given me, I readily agreed. I had been informed of the potential problems, the fact that it may not be successful, and all of the risks. The recovery from the surgery was very painful, but I quickly returned to good health and have been making great physical strides since then. I did not experience any stress from having the surgery.

It has been a little over two years from the date of the surgery, and I have lost the weight I gained. Currently, the MG does not affect my physical activity, and I exercise daily again and feel great. I currently do not have any problems with fatigue, difficulty swallowing, slurring of speech, or diplopia. I do not feel the MG affected me psychologically, except it made me determined to overcome this problem and enjoy life. I still am on a low dosage of prednisone, but I am able to cope with the hunger and make myself control my appetite. I have routine bone-density tests and continue to take calcium regularly. I did not receive IVIG or plasma exchange.

My advice to those who must face this trial is to stay positive. You can beat it. I was fortunate to have a wonderful family to support me and encourage me every step of the way. Let your friends and family help you and thank them for what they do.

> *"My advice to those who must face this
> trial is to stay positive. You can beat it."*

## Expert Comment:

Patients may ask "Why me?" MG does not recognize borders and can affect anyone. It is more common in middle-aged women and older men, but even children can be affected. Do not blame yourself.

When MG goes into remission, medications should not be discontinued.

There is no universal protocol, but if the disease is in complete remission (no symptoms) for two years, the physician may decide to very slowly taper the medications. Of course, relapse is still possible, but less than with an early discontinuation.

Patients may be shocked when they are given the diagnosis for the first time, especially if they were leading a very healthy and athletic life. Yes, MG may limit the extent of physical activity, but most patients will be able to engage in activities needed for an average lifestyle.

It is important that the surgeon and anesthesiologist know about your disease so that they avoid certain anesthetics and medications. Communications between them and the treating physician should always be open.

Thymectomy can be painful. Increasingly, minimally invasive thymectomy is becoming more available and mastered by some thoracic surgeons, and it is becoming more acceptable by neuromuscular specialists after years of hesitation because of the possibility of inaccessibility of all the thymus gland to resection. This possibility is important in rare cases where the thymus has ramifications or ectopic satellites that would make even open surgery difficult. For tumor resection, open thymectomy with sternal split is still the recommended modality.

Staying positive throughout the treatment period is very important. Anxiety and depression may be exacerbated by steroids, and some patients may need antidepressants. Anxiety attacks may be confused with myasthenic crisis, as fatigue and shortness of breath are common to both. This may lead to increasing the dose of the MG medications or institution of more aggressive treatments like IVIG or PLEX unnecessarily. Ironically, anxiety symptoms may well improve with these interventions, enforcing the notion that the symptoms were due to MG. Experience is needed to make these decisions.

> *"Experience is needed to treat MG."*

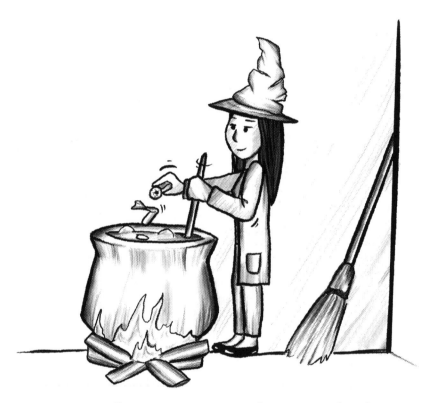

Virgin fly wing, tears of a neurologist,
And I made a steroid potion.

# Case #38

## MYASTHENIA GRAVIS: MY CHALLENGES AND JOURNEY TO A NORMAL LIFE

"Decreased visual acuity is not a feature of MG
but of an eye disease like cataracts..."

My father's family has always had a history of declining eyesight health. I have a brother and an aunt who have macular degeneration to the degree that both are now legally blind. Naturally, I developed a concern that this declining eye health could one day hit me and often thought about *What would I do if I were to go blind? How much of God's beautiful creation would I miss if I did? How awful would it be if I could not lay eyes on my beautiful wife again?* This thought process was one of the driving forces behind my desire to travel and see more of God's beautiful world with my God-given spouse.

This concern about vision loss manifested itself when I suddenly had the onset of double vision. Now, not only was I seeing the beauty of the world, but I was seeing it twice ... at the same time. Immediately, my life changed. I prayed to God about losing my vision and asked Him to guide me to a place where I could get the medical attention I needed.

My optometrist advised me to go to one of the top ophthalmologists in another state. After a full day of testing on my eyes, it was somewhat comforting to know that I did not have macular degeneration. However, the eye clinic could not resolve my issues, and I was referred by the ophthalmologist to the neurologist who is my current doctor. Numerous questions crossed my mind, such as, *Okay, God, if the top eye ophthalmology clinic out of town cannot resolve my double-vision issues, what else could there be?* This first thought process was a fear of the unknown. Then I just gave in to a peace that only Jesus Himself can render and put my trust in Him by following through on the appointment.

Fortunately, the doctor was able to see me (and I saw my doctor twice … at the same time) very first thing the following day. My son drove me to the doctor's office, as his single vision was far safer than my double, accident-prone vision on the drive out of town. My son is a registered nurse. Although he was driving me to the doctor's office, I may have approached the edge of driving my son to the brink of insanity. He was inundated with a multitude of questions regarding what could be causing this double vision. My son's professional, well-rehearsed nurse's response was to "just wait and see what the doctor says." Good nurse … great son.

When I arrived at the doctor's office, I noticed a plaque on the wall where he was voted as one of the top 100 physicians in the United States by the American Medical Board. That gave me some comfort. Even with that knowledge, though, the question still in my head was, *What is my problem?* Fearful of what the answer might be, I resolved to rely on my strong belief in God to see me through all of the challenges that might lie ahead.

The short amount of time I spent in the waiting room seemed like an eternity, although it was less than ten minutes. Thoughts like *Why send me to a neurologist?* and *Is my problem worse than just going blind?* had me operating out of my comfort zone. Throughout this whole process, I had to remind myself that God is in control, and whatever lies ahead I have a living God who will see me through it all.

The long wait (ten minutes or less) finally was over when my doctor met me at the door. Immediately, he looked into my eyes and just stated, "Yes … myasthenia gravis," without any test to even verify what was wrong. My immediate thoughts were, *How does he know without any testing?* and *What the heck is myasthenia gravis?* After a brief explanation of what he thought it was, which was verified with subsequent testing, I felt like a weight had been lifted off of my shoulders. Truly, God had put me in the path of my current doctor who was extremely knowledgeable in the subject matter and was able to provide me with a peace about my life and my future.

> *"Now, not only was I seeing the beauty of the world, but I was seeing it twice at the same time."*

My doctor said that droopy eyes are the first indicator of myasthenia gravis. I had that Bluetick Hound kind of droopiness, so my doctor could tell just by looking in my eyes what the issue was. The first of many subsequent questions was answered.

My doctor provided me with a prescription of a high level of prednisone, pyridostigmine, and azathioprine, along with over-the-counter Pepcid AC and 1,200 mg/day of calcium. Within a week, my vision had returned to normal, but I now had a voracious appetite. Being from the South, I had a constant craving for crawfish and beef, with a lot of cakes, cookies, ice cream, and anything else I could get my hands on to eat. Along with the eating came a constant thirst that I originally quenched with an abundance of Diet Coke.

With the excessive eating and drinking habit I developed from the high dosage of prednisone and the poor selection of food groups, I gained approximately eighty pounds. In addition, whatever liquid goes in eventually has to come out. I found at the elevated levels of prednisone, I had lost my ability to actually hold my bladder long enough to make it to the restroom many times. I got into the habit of always bringing spare pants and underwear to change into when those embarrassing moments came.

I was on the verge of wondering now if my life was going to be a life of living in Depends, and darn … I felt I was way too young for that. My inability to have single vision was now replaced by my inability to control my bladder long enough to get to the restroom. Thankfully, this side effect was short-lived as well. A change in my diet plan (or lack of planning) and stopping the constant infusion of the diuretic Diet Coke, combined with lower levels of prednisone for the maintenance dosage, brought this constant bathroom marathon to an end.

Further testing revealed that my hemoglobin A1C had shot up to 6.3 percent. In layman's terms, I now had borderline type 2 diabetes. That resulted in additional medication to combat the diabetes and a need to make a change in my diet plan. I found out through my nutritionist wife that cookies and Little Debbie cakes were not a good source of fiber, and that ice cream (although made with milk and eggs) was not a good source of protein and calcium. With the coaching and encouragement of my wife (who does hold a master's degree in nutrition), I began to change those self-destructive habits to achieve a healthier nutrition plan.

In addition, my prednisone dosage began to decrease, and the excessive cravings subsided. I am now on a healthy diet and well on my way to losing the weight, with a goal to achieve my pre-MG weight. With this change, my A1C, which is a measure of where you stand in the world of diabetes, is being well controlled, and I am now out of the threat zone of prediabetes.

Follow-up visits with my doctor, continuous monitoring of the MG, the impacts of the medicine, and overall neurological help has kept me on a path of controlling the disease. This has included changes in medication (including significant reductions in my prednisone usage), bone-density testing, and monthly blood work. However, due to my job, I have not been able to keep up with the monthly blood work that is required of me. In my employment, I do an extensive amount of travel. Much of this travel takes me to places where I cannot obtain the blood work that my doctor would like to see on a regular basis.

I have had to discipline myself to go to the laboratories to have my blood work completed and sent to my doctor every time I am in town and the blood work is due. This is a critical part of the overall treatment plan, and without this, my doctor does not have all of the information he needs to continue optimizing my treatment plan. Bottom line, regardless of how busy my employment keeps me, the regular laboratory test is a critical part of the overall treatment plan.

An integral part of optimizing my medical treatment plan was the reduction of prednisone. This had to be reduced to a point of double-vision relapse. Unfortunately, I was out of town when the optimization had achieved its limit and I began again to have double vision. A call was made to my doctor's office regarding this. Unfortunately, my doctor was out of town at the time, and the phone tag with his office with a backup physician's failure to contact me resulted in my making a semi-educated decision on my own. I increased the dosage of my prednisone slightly. I had carried only a week's supply of medicine with me on this particular trip, so I was having to rob some of the prednisone from days later in the week to help regain my single vision.

Another route I took was the use of an eye patch. I was able to cover one eye and reduce the vision to single vision. Upon returning to my doctor's office, I was able to discuss this incident with my doctor. I was informed that the next time this happened and I was unable to reach him, I should increase my pyridostigmine instead of the prednisone. Although my self-medication worked, it was not the best route to take. I now carry additional pyridostigmine in my medication supply for out-of-town trips. The eye patch also helped to maintain a single-vision perception, although it was quite annoying.

> *"An eye patch is a very useful trick to correct double vision."*

My background is a doctorate in physical chemistry. As such, I have a thorough understanding of reaction mechanisms of various chemistries when you combine them. Even with this knowledge, however, I did not know the formulations of some of the pharmaceuticals that I was taking without further research. I therefore obtained a list of these chemistries and a list from my doctor as to what medications either had a reaction with my MG medications or had a negative impact on the symptoms of MG. I have insured that each of the doctors I go to, including my family doctor, cardiologist, pulmonologist, and any other *-ologist* that I may encounter, has that list in my medical records, which can be used as a quick reference when they write me miscellaneous prescriptions.

Fortunately, with the medical plan that my doctor has set up for me, I have had no restrictions in my physical activities. I do get tired after walking five to ten miles per day, but I attribute that to either getting older or realizing that *You know … five to ten miles of walking per day is a pretty good walk*. In summary, the treatment protocol that my doctor has set up for me, the leadership of my nutritionist wife, the general counsel of my nurse son, and the encouragement of all those around me has aided me in living a life that is rich and full. With the power of God alive in me, I am thankful for His guidance for me to meet my doctor, who in my case was indeed a miracle worker.

> *"My doctor was a miracle worker."*

**Expert Comment:**

Decreased visual acuity is not a feature of MG but of an eye disease like cataracts, glaucoma, and retinal disorders. Blurring of vision is usually due to steroids and less commonly due to MG. Although double vision is the classical feature of MG, it can be caused by many factors that may affect the functions of the eye muscles and nerves, including brain tumor and muscular dystrophy. Risk of cataract and glaucoma is increased by chronic steroid therapy.

An annual eye examination is recommended for all myasthenics to check on these possibilities. Double vision can be dangerous, especially during driving. An eye patch is a reasonable temporary solution. Seeing beauty twice is good, but not all patients are happy to see their doctors twice.

Urinary incontinence is not a feature of MG. However, ladies with stress incontinence or males who have had prostate surgery may rely on their external sphincter to hold their urine as the internal sphincter is weakened. The internal sphincter is made of smooth muscles that are not affected by MG, but the external sphincter is made of a skeletal muscle that *is* affected by MG. Therefore, urinary incontinence may happen in severe cases of MG. That said, incontinence should be evaluated by a urologist to rule out other causes.

Bone density may be reduced by chronic steroid therapy, rendering bones softer and increasing the risk of fractures with even minimal falls. Therefore, calcium and vitamin D are always recommended with steroid therapy in addition to an annual bone-density scan to detect and treat osteoporosis early. Maintaining physical activity is important to keep the bone alive.

Travel policy for myasthenics is an important part of treatment. It is not recommended that patients travel in the beginning of treatment and while on high-dose steroids because their body is weak, fatigue is common, and the stress of travel may create problems. Also, it is not recommended to travel during tapering of medications due to increased risk of relapse. However, once the patient is on a stable dose of medications, travel would be allowed. It is important for the treating physician to know about your travel plan to provide you with a number to call for emergencies and with phone numbers of myasthenia specialists in the state or country you are visiting. You may visit the website of the myasthenia gravis foundation of America (MGFA) for a list of MG-treating physicians in the United States.

Monthly blood testing is important to check for side effects of some medications like azathioprine and methotrexate. Normally, blood count and what are called *liver enzymes* are checked. Some patients do not take this seriously, and their negative reaction to the medicine is not detected early. They may become prone to infection, and their liver function may deteriorate, which they will only know after being admitted to the hospital. These tests can be done even in remote areas and abroad and should not be overlooked. Sometimes, more or less frequent testing is ordered depending on the case.

> **"What are the travel guidelines for myasthenics?"**

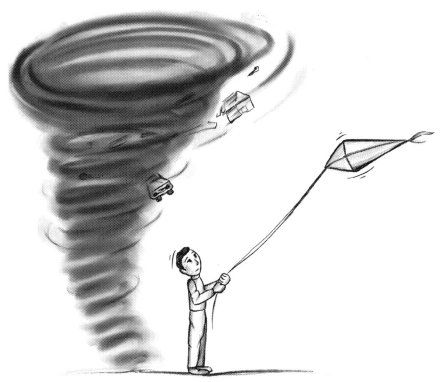

Best wind for kite flying is a hurricane

# Case #39

## I'm a Believer in Living with Whatever I Have

"I used to jump out of airplanes, and now I can't even jump out of bed. I have accepted that fact."

One day, I was driving my limousine at night to pick up a customer. As I was heading from the airport to the hotel, all I could see was screeching red lights. I had to close one eye, and that's how I had to drive. I dropped my customer off and went home, all while using just one eye.

Then, the next morning, one of my eyelids just closed shut, and I couldn't open it. I tried to use force to open it, but it was difficult. I decided to go see my eye doctor. Once I got an appointment with my eye doctor, she said I had myasthenia gravis. She tried to help me by putting thicker glasses on and checking me out. But it wasn't helping. One of my eyelids opened and the other one closed.

I was having a lot of trouble with my eyes, and at this point I couldn't drive. She told me I had to go see a neurologist, because I had a strong case of MG and she couldn't straighten my eyesight out. That's when I went to see a neurologist. The neurologist said he couldn't do anything because he knew very little about the disease, and there were very few neurologists who knew about it, let alone would work with it. So that neurologist sent me to see a myasthenia gravis specialist.

I went to see the specialist, and he told me what was going on. I reacted to the diagnosis like anybody else would. I was thinking, *What's going on? Why me? What happened?* It was human nature. But I thought to myself, *I'm in my seventies, and stuff like this just happens.* So I've learned to accept it.

All I know how to do is drive a truck, since I drive for a living. I have had a lot of odd hours of sleeping. Sometimes I would sleep during the day, sometimes at night, sometimes two, three hours then back on a truck and drive, so my job caused quite a bit of stress on my eyes and body. I believe that's how this happened.

The first medication the doctor put me on that year was pyridostigmine bromide. At the time, I refused to take prednisone; I had heard so many bad things about steroids, I said I didn't want to take anything of the sort. After about a year of seeing this specialist, he said, "You're going on prednisone, because the pyridostigmine is not working."

That was a shocker, because I'm a diabetic with high blood pressure. There were a lot of reasons I didn't want to take steroids, and one of them was because I had my diabetes under control through exercise and eating right. Prednisone messed with my blood pressure and blood sugar. My blood pressure went so high, and my sugar was up to 600. I couldn't control it. So I went to the emergency room, and all my doctors were in communication with the specialist. They were asking him why he had me on such a heavy dose, but all he said was they needed to work around him. So I had to keep taking it!

Then they finally put me on insulin, which I didn't want to do either, since I'm not very fond of any medication. While waiting for the prednisone to kick in, I dealt with the double vision by closing one eye and by using an eye patch. I kept switching the eye patch back and forth between both eyes, and I did this technique for a couple of months to try to straighten the eyes.

In about a month I started seeing positive effects from the steroids, and my symptoms started improving. My eyesight in the beginning was still a little disrupted, and it was blurry at times, but it was helping. However, soon after, the double vision was straightening out, and then I stopped having double vision. I no longer needed to use the eye patch.

The neurologist tapered me off down from 80 mg to what I'm taking now, which is 15 mg. To this day I'm still under his care.

> **"Prednisone drove my blood sugar up to 600mg/dl and I had to be placed on insulin."**

I didn't have any bad side effects with the pyridostigmine. It was kind of helping me, but it was not straightening my eyesight out. When I was on pyridostigmine, the double vision stayed with me for that full year, so that's when the doctor decided to switch me to prednisone. I didn't see any benefits to the prednisone other than it straightening my eyes out. I did notice that some of the medications caused me to swell up, especially with all the adjustments in the medication plan. He would taper me off and put me on another medication.

My cardiologist had to take me off some pills that were really causing me to swell up, especially in my legs. So I tried to work with that. Also, I think the medication caused me to have some swallowing difficulties, because before the medication I didn't have any. But, as he began to taper me off the steroids, the swallowing difficulties subsided, and I'm doing a lot better.

Between the time I was diagnosed with MG and now, I had a stent put in, but I have that under control. I'm seventy-six, so what else can I do? At one point in my life, I also had colon cancer, and I survived. Luckily, that's under control. I also make sure to get my colonoscopies, and every time I come out clear for that as well. To be cautious, whenever I go to see another doctor, I always show a list of medications I am currently taking and medications to avoid that was given to me by the MG doctor. I keep all my doctors in communication with each other.

I go to my cardiologist to get a checkup every three to six months and he says everything looks good. Normally, I watch what I eat, and I try to exercise every day or at least three to four times a week. I do this to keep my sugar and blood pressure under control. In the morning, I go do some cardio and a little bit of resistance. Then, when I come back, I eat breakfast and I take my medication. There is the occasional time when I go overboard on a few things I eat and drink, I like my beer, and sometimes I slack off on my exercising, but overall I try to keep a healthy diet. I make sure to monitor my sugar and take insulin when I need it because when I indulge, I know my blood pressure and sugar goes up, so I try to do it in moderation.

For example, this weekend, we went to an Eagles concert with all the kids. One of my sons rented one of those suites. So of course, we had food and beverages, and I kind of overdid it because my kids were here from out of town. But now I am back to reality.

Before I started taking the medication, the MG really didn't affect my ability to exercise, but I was so busy working all the time that I really didn't notice if it did affect me. I still pushed myself to exercise. When I was first taking a heavy dose of steroids, it did affect my ability to exercise, but now that I am on 15 mg, I push myself. Of course, I get a little tired on the days that I take it, but I know I have to push myself. The work is strenuous, but like I said, it's something that I have to overpower. I just accept the fact that this is what I have to do.

I notice that at times when I'm completely tired, I will have a relapse in symptoms. Especially at night, I start feeling the effects of the MG. I just close my eyes and lie down, and next morning I'm okay.

I'm not a believer in dying of anything. I'm a believer in living with whatever I have. I have MG, and I'm going to live with it. I'm not going to die from it.

Of course, MG affected me psychologically, especially in the beginning. Like I said earlier, everybody goes through the "why me." But not anymore. I have accepted it. I look around and for a seventy-six-year-old man, I'm doing better than a lot of fifty-year-olds and sixty-year-olds. I understand that I can't do the things I used to do, and that's okay. I used to jump out of airplanes, and now I can't even jump out of bed. I have accepted that fact. I've realized that people want to die of something, but I don't. I want to live with something. It doesn't matter what—I am going to live through it!

I try not to be a negative person. I don't like to look at the things going wrong. I look at how I'm improving. I'm not going to let something control my mental state. It's like I always say: stop thinking of the negative part of what you have. There's a lot of things that I can't do that I used to be able to do, but I'm not going to let it ruin me. I refuse to get up in the morning and say, "Why me? What did I do to deserve this?"

Try to accept the fact that this is the hand you were dealt. Live with it; don't die with it, and don't die of it. Continue to live, and if you have to change your life around it, well then, you just have to change.

> **"I have MG, and I'm going to live with it. I'm not going to die from it."**

**Expert Comment:**

MG may force a change of lifestyle and is not compatible with certain professions. Truck driving is one of those professions that rely on vision for life. It is important to avoid driving with double vision. This is more so in the second half of the day. An eye patch or a prism may provide temporarily relief but isn't totally safe, as depth and peripheral vision are needed.

Blood sugar and blood pressure go up most of the time with steroid treatment. Patients, especially diabetics and hypertensives, need to check their blood sugar and blood pressure several times daily and communicate with their primary-care physician or cardiologist to treat these conditions by starting or adjusting medications. Patients should not wait until they go to the ER to be told that their blood sugar is 600. Most of the time, when the steroid dose is tapered, these symptoms will improve, and those who become diabetic will not be anymore.

Pharmacies and other specialists who are not familiar with MG often are surprised by the dose of prednisone. Patients may get alarmed by their comments. They should not change the dose of the medication without consulting with the treating physician. On the other hand, pharmacists may discover an interaction that the treating physician is not aware of. They may provide useful input to the treating physician.

Communication among all physicians treating the patient is very important to avoid worsening other conditions while treating MG. We recommend that a clinical note be provided to the patient to share with other physicians, and that a note be faxed to the main treating physicians.

The effect of alcoholic beverages on MG and its treatment is a common concern. Light consumption of alcohol, such as a glass of wine a day away from the dosing time of the medications, is usually not associated with worsening of the MG and usually does not interact with its medications. However, heavy consumption of alcohol may worsen the fatigue, accentuate the ill effect of the steroids on the stomach, and interfere with sleep.

> **"Communication among all physicians treating the patient is very important."**

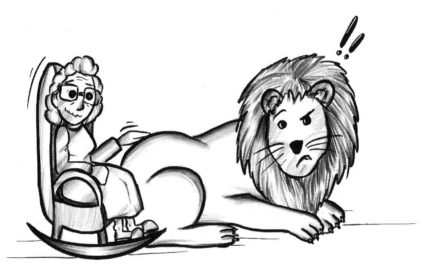

Are you eating my steroid again Lily?

# Case #40

## NEVER ACCEPT AGE AS THE CAUSE OF DOUBLE VISION

Little did I know that on October 16, 2014, my sight was on the road to recovery, thanks to my doctor. As my daughter looked at me, I knew it was even more serious than I had imagined. My eyesight issue was obviously very visible to others. She exclaimed, "Oh, Mother, what is wrong with your eyes? They are each moving in different directions!"

I had been experiencing double vision all week, and as an avid reader of my King James Holy Bible, I had been unable to focus on the words. In fact, it was even impossible now to drive or even watch my favorite TV shows, all due to this double vision I was experiencing. I was sixty-nine years young, still taking annual road trips with my husband to visit our great nation's national parks, being active in our church, and occasionally driving to the local grocery store or nail and beauty salon.

My new husband and I lived four hundred miles away from my daughter, and she was visiting us at the time. Earlier in the week, I had gone to see my eye doctor of forty-plus years, whose office was several hundred miles away. He had announced, "This is just weak eye muscles due to your rapidly declining age, and you will just have to live with it." As frightening as that diagnosis was, he was the doctor, and I trusted him, so I accepted that diagnosis.

However, when I told my daughter, she googled "causes of eyes moving separately and double vision" and came up with several possibilities. She refused to accept that this was just something I had to live with. Thus began the task of calling and visiting doctors.

Just prior to my vision doubling and losing control of my eyes, I had experienced major heart surgery. Over the next six weeks, I saw another eye doctor and two medical doctors. Finally, I was referred to my new doctor, the angel we had been praying for, who quickly diagnosed and began treating my symptoms. Thankfully, the pronunciation of my diagnosis, myasthenia gravis, would be much more difficult than the actual treatment.

However, the side effects of taking 80 mg of prednisone daily (with an added 600 units three times a day of vitamin D) would drastically change my appearance, which I had not prepared myself for, even though my doctor had warned me of this. My face doubled in size, and as an already overweight senior, I found myself wearing muumuu dresses and not wanting to go out in public due to my distorted facial appearance and symptoms of diarrhea followed by bouts of depression. But I would change nothing, for I had regained my sight and active lifestyle.

Today, I am down to 10 mg every other day and have no swelling or noticeable side effects. I maintain my vitamin D regimen, which all seniors should follow. God bless my doctor and all the kind staff who helped to restore my sight.

> *"Thankfully, the pronunciation of my diagnosis, myasthenia gravis, would be much more difficult than the actual treatment."*

**Expert Comment:**

The diagnosis of MG is usually delayed due to subtlety of symptoms and lack of experience. There is nothing wrong with seeking a second opinion if the patient is not satisfied with an answer.

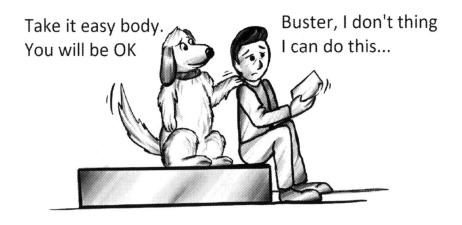

# Case #41

## No Success Story to Tell Yet

"Weakness of the neck extensors is an uncommon but a certain feature of MG."

My earliest symptoms were weakness in my legs and double vision. My diagnosis came three years later. I got glasses with a prism in one lens so I could drive and watch movies. When I was first diagnosed, I was happy to finally receive a diagnosis, because I assumed that meant treatment was available.

The first treatment given by the doctor was Mestinon, which gave me no relief, and the side effects were unacceptable. The second treatment I received was prednisone, which again, I received no relief from, and the side effects I experienced were weight gain and dry mouth. These are the only treatments I have received, and I have had no other treatment yet.

I changed my dosage of the steroid on my own, but I went back to a doctor-planned weaning off process. I received a list of medications not to take from my doctor, and whenever I was prescribed a new medication, I would call the doctor to verify if I could take it.

I am not sure if myasthenia gravis has affected my daily physical activity. I do feel very weak, but I cannot be sure if that is totally a result of MG. I have not exercised at all. I do have fatigue that has not been dealt with. I do not know how to cope with it, and it has been very difficult. The double vision has also been very difficult. I use special glasses at the moment.

Having myasthenia gravis has definitely affected me psychologically. On occasion, when the symptoms are affecting me adversely, I do get depressed. I find playing with my dog cheers me up. He should probably be an emotional support dog.

The steroids adversely affected my weight. I had been on steroids before and gained a lot of weight, so when I went on the steroids again, my weight once again started to go up. In terms of advice, I have not had success in battling this illness, so I don't have any advice.

> *"When I am depressed from steroids, my dog cheers me up. He is my support."*

**Expert Comment:**

The most common cause of steroid failure is inadequate dose or duration or premature tapering due to side effects or lack of experience. Lack of response to adequate dose and duration of prednisone occurs in less than 10 percent of cases. One has to revisit the diagnosis before moving to a more aggressive regimen.

There are many causes of diplopia and leg weakness that should be investigated. Leg weakness is not uncommon in MG, and it can be the presenting symptom in a minority of cases, imposing a diagnostic difficulty. If other causes are excluded and/or MG is confirmed, other lines of treatment may include chemotherapy (azathioprine, methotrexate, cyclosporin, etc.), intravenous gamma globulin, plasma exchange, and rituximab. It may take several months of treatment to see a response.

Sometimes, an offensive drug needs to be excluded, such as ciprofloxacin, streptomycin, or quinine. A latent infection may cause MG to be refractory. Thymoma is another possible reason. It is important to identify the symptoms that are expected to respond to treatment in order to know what to expect.

Some patients think that leg pain, back pain, feet numbness, dizziness, or fatigue due to sleep apnea will get better, and since these symptoms are not related to MG, they will not change. Sometimes they may get worse, such as sleep apnea and blurring of vision. Also, sometimes what looks like ptosis is in fact a droopy forehead skin (dermatochalasis).

> *"The most common cause of steroid failure is inadequate dose or duration or premature tapering due to side effects or lack of experience."*

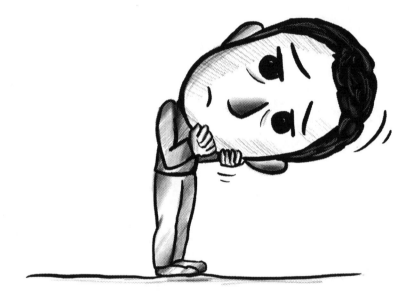

I think this disease is getting into my head!

# Case #42

## I Could Not Raise My Head

> "I'm weak and worn out and upset, but my doctor
> keeps telling me that I'm doing great."

At the end of February 2018, I woke up one morning seeing double. I was freaked out, wondering what was going on, I didn't know what to think. I was upset, unhappy, and worried all at the same time.

I noticed that if I closed one eye, I could see normally. So I went to work anyway, assuming this problem was temporary and that it would soon go away. But it didn't, so after two or three days, I decided to go to an eye doctor and get it checked. They gave me some eye drops and sent me home.

Two more days went by, and still nothing improved. I went back to the eye doctor, who told me to go to a specialist. I made an appointment with a specialist and went a couple of days later, and that doctor sent me to another specialist. This specialist did some tests and told me he would let me know something when he got back from vacation.

Approximately two weeks later, he called and told me I had myasthenia gravis. He recommended me to someone who specialized in MG. During the two-week wait for test results, in two days, I lost control of my neck. Because of this, I would just swing my head back so I could still drive.

When I got the results, I was happy, because the situation was kind of scary—especially three or four of those days during the two-week wait when my eyelids would droop. First the double vision, then my neck would start falling because I couldn't hold my head up straight, and lastly, my eyes started drooping. I was really feeling terrible.

My doctor immediately put me on prednisone, and within two weeks, the weakness disappeared and has never returned. Thank God and my doctor for helping me to continue working. It's been two years, and I feel great. I have not had any problems with any medication as of yet. I have not had a thymectomy, and I have not tried changing the dose of the medications. I have followed the specialist's orders since the beginning.

> *"My neck muscles were so weak, that I could not lift my head to see ahead. I spotted a lot of money on the ground."*

**Expert Comment:**

Weakness of the neck extensors (the muscles that lift the head) is an uncommon but a certain feature of MG. It can be part of a generalized picture, but it may be the presenting feature. It usually causes social embarrassment and functional impairment. The patient cannot hold his or her head, so that some use their hands to do so. The weakness worsens in the evening, and it becomes hard to watch TV. Pain in the back of the neck is common due to strain of the neck muscles.

There are eight pairs of muscles that lift the head up. They are located in the back of the neck. Patients who have this as the only feature of MG may be suspected of having a cervical spine problem, especially if the MRI of the cervical spine shows some degenerative changes. But cervical spine changes do not cause dropped head.

There are other causes of dropped head that need to be considered, such as a muscle disease called *axial myopathy* where the paraspinal muscles are affected by muscle disease. Lou Gehrig's disease may also present with dropped head. If double vision and ptosis are present, then the diagnosis of MG will become easier. Sometimes blood and other testing are negative, and the only option is to treat as a case of MG and wait for a response.

> *"Dropped head can be caused by MG and other neuromuscular disorders such as ALS."*

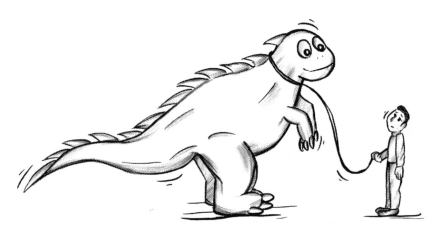

Can you do tricks?

# Case #43

## Get a Pet

"This was not the way I planned to spend my retirement."

At first I noticed something was wrong because I was getting weaker and weaker, and it was getting harder and harder to walk. I had no stamina and was breathing hard; I was trying to get from the parking lot to the hospital where I was working. I was also having trouble chewing and swallowing, and I couldn't get around like I used to.

The swallowing difficulties were so intense that I was basically living on a liquid diet at one point. This is because every time I chewed something and tried to swallow it, it'd go down the wrong way and into my lungs. So I couldn't eat solids. Strictly ingesting liquids caused me to lose a lot of weight. This wasn't a bad thing for me, because at that time, I was in the 300s.

Anyway, I remember going to Disney World, and I'm bopping around on a scooter going to a restaurant with my family. but I couldn't eat. I ordered a chicken noodle soup, and all I could do was sip the broth.

I didn't go to see a doctor, and my symptoms just kept getting worse and worse until finally it hit a point where I couldn't function. I had to stop like three to four times in the morning just to get from my car to the hospital. Then chewing and swallowing became more difficult. So I just said to heck with it, and I went to see my primary-care physician (PCP).

The doctor gave me a quick run over and referred me to a neurologist for a consultation. The appointment was maybe a week or two weeks from seeing my PCP. I went to see the neurologist, and the neurologist gave me a quick check and then an in-depth physical exam, as well as some blood work. I got called back within two days, and he told me the blood work said I had myasthenia gravis. He then referred me to a specialist in the field.

When the doctor said I had myasthenia gravis, I wasn't exactly sure what it was. Other than having trouble swallowing and being kind of weak, I wasn't feeling all that bad. When I went to see an MG specialist, we went over all the information about the disease, and that was about it. I didn't get warm fuzzy feelings from the doctor.

There was an additional neurologist they sent me to who seemed like a nice guy. But the specialist I saw was so cold toward me. I felt like he was more concerned with other stuff than he was concerned about me. I feel that way every time.

Anyway, I'm diabetic and have been for years. My diabetes has been controlled by staying away from sugar and taking my medication. My MG doctor put me on these massive doses of steroids, and my sugar went through the ever-loving roof. I told him, "Man, this stuff is messing with my sugar. Why am I going through all these things?"

His response was, "That's okay. That's what the insulin is for."

I felt like he just blew it off, like he didn't seem to care. I had to remind him that I was a diabetic and my sugar was running into the 400s. What did he mean that it wasn't important?

Later, the doctor talked me into a thymectomy because it seemed to help slow down the progress of the disease. I wasn't exactly crazy about the idea because I'd had surgeries before, and I wasn't crazy about them. But I finally agreed and had the procedure done. Let me tell you, I have never had a recovery from surgery as bad as this one. Once I got out of the hospital, I noticed that every time I coughed, sneezed, or moved, my chest would hurt like crazy.

Anyway, I got done with that, but I kept getting weaker and weaker. Even now, my knees and my legs are killing me when I walk. Even getting from the couch to the bathroom just wipes me out. I'm weak and worn out and upset, but my doctor keeps telling me that I'm doing great.

> ### *"The swallowing difficulties were so intense that I was basically living on a liquid diet at one point."*

I am not sure if the thymectomy helped or not. My doctor says that the surgery has helped me a whole lot, which could be possible, but I am not sure. I understand my condition could be worse, and without the thymectomy, it probably would have been worse. I was sixty-two when I was diagnosed, and I am now sixty-six. So the surgery probably has slowed things down a lot in the last four years, from what I have read about the disease.

However, I don't feel support and comfort from my doctors, so my outlook and feelings on the situation aren't positive. The doctor said he is cutting down my steroids to 15 milligrams every other day. At this point, I've gotten used to taking the insulin, and my sugar is under control, but I'm just not a happy camper.

I used to take large doses of steroids when my asthma would act up, but the steroids would make me feel so sick. The steroids I was given for my asthma are nowhere near as bad as the ones for my MG. The steroids made me hungry and mean. So you can imagine my poor family when I'm getting these large doses of steroids. It was not just affecting me but everybody around me. The steroids just made me act so horribly. I was always having to apologize to the people around me and explain that it wasn't me but the medication.

I couldn't find a good way to control my emotions or how I was feeling while taking these large doses of medication, other than to just apologize and explain my situation. It only started to get better once the steroids were tapered down. My sugar was under control, and so were my emotions and appetite.

I did have a bad relapse with my MG one time and ended up in the hospital. I was there for about three weeks, and they gave me a whole bunch of medications. One of the medications they gave me was called azathioprine, which I heard is a type of chemotherapy drug. I currently take the medication three times per day, and it does help my symptoms a lot.

I have always tried to stick to the doctor's plan as best I could and never tried to change the dosing. Even though I was difficult, I always listened and followed orders. I also made sure that I gave all my doctors lists of the medications I was taking so they would know. Also, my pharmacist went through the list and made sure that none of the drugs I was being prescribed would interact with my MG medicine.

> ## *"I couldn't find a good way to control my emotions."*

I also have asthma, and when I first got diagnosed, I didn't want to let it control me. But I did struggle with it, and a couple of times it has sent me to the emergency room and ICU. I didn't want to take the situation lightly. After that, I started paying attention to my symptoms, and I began taking my medications properly and started carrying my inhalers everywhere.

With myasthenia gravis, I wanted to do the same thing, so I started paying more attention to it. I heard you were supposed to take an afternoon nap and go to bed early, but that didn't go with my work ethic. I should probably get more rest, because I do start to get tired during the day. A couple of times, I have broken down and taken a nap, and I did feel better. But if I sleep in for too long, then I can't go to sleep at night, so I don't know what to do.

This was not the way I planned to spend my retirement. I wasn't planning on retiring this early. I planned on working until I was at least sixty-five or sixty-seven years old, but I had to retire at sixty-two. Now, I sit on the couch, eat, sleep, and go to the bathroom. I don't have the strength to go anywhere else. I can't go to family parties or gatherings because I don't have the strength, and transporting me there is a big production. It's like taking a newborn baby to see Grandma and Grandpa—all that stuff you must pack up and haul around. That's me. I feel bad sometimes, and I'm just angry, so I try to vent, but I feel like people think I am getting mad at them.

I didn't expect to get better, because, like I said, I didn't know much about the disease. You might have times when things aren't all that bad, but then you hit plateaus. I just know I'm not going to get any better, and I know things are going to start getting worse.

I also feel like dealing with this situation has messed with my mental health. I started off with some anger issues. I used to get mad and blow up at times. I do think I have a little bit of PTSD. I've never had it diagnosed or anything, but I think I have it. I used to be a medic in the Air Force back in the day. I was stationed out on an island close to the North Atlantic for a year and a half. I was exposed to a severely traumatic situation. So I think I have some PTSD from my time there. I think that's why I get these anger issues all the time, and I think my diagnosis with MG made it worse.

Luckily, my anger is not as bad as it used to be. I'm getting older, and I'm mellowing out in my old age. But I am angry about this situation, God, and the world. I don't know why God did this to me. I understand I'm not exactly an angel; I never have been. I'm not the nicest guy in the world, but I don't think I deserve this.

The anger comes in stages. I get angry, I calm down, and it happens all over again. However, I feel like my wife and family have helped me a lot when it comes to my mood and how I feel. I wouldn't be able to cope without them. I believe that how I am feeling is a part of the grieving process. Currently, I'm at the angry stage.

Myasthenia gravis has also affected my physical activity. I can't exercise like I used to, not like I did much anyway. For a while, I went to see a nutritionist who put me on a diet and told me to start exercising, so I started watching fitness videos. For a while there, when I first started, it was awfully hard to work out because I was really weak. So lately, I haven't been doing it. That's why I decided to quit.

When I was first diagnosed and newly retired, I was still in good enough shape that I was able to get around with just a cane. I was still able to get out by myself. I used to pick up my granddaughter from school in the afternoon and go to the grocery store or junk shops, but I can't do that now. Now, I can't get around with just the cane; I need a walker. Nobody lets me drive, so I'm stuck in the house, and I have to depend on people to take me places. I used to be able to get out and take little trips by myself. I can't do that anymore.

To this day, after all the medications, I still suffer from cramps in my hands and my legs. I don't know if that's MG or just me having cramps. My fingers tingle all the time and are a bit numb, but I think that's from the diabetes. I don't have strength in my knees and legs. It hurts to walk, but I am not sure if that's the arthritis or the MG. I just don't have any strength and stamina anymore.

Sometimes, to this day, I still have difficulty swallowing, and I have to slow down my eating and drinking. For example, when I swallow my pills, I have to take them one or two at a time. In the old days, I used to be able to take a bunch of pills at the same time with no problem, but I can't do that anymore. So to help me swallow, I just do a little at a time and make sure to swallow slowly.

Having this disease is hard. It makes you angry, it makes you sad, but you've got to count your blessings, because no matter how bad it is, it can be worse. I used to work at the VA (Veterans Affairs), and I used to see guys who were in really bad shape. You would see guys lying in bed who couldn't talk, couldn't move, and were fed through tubes. Then you would see other guys who were getting around in wheelchairs. They could sit up, and all you would hear them talking about is how sick they were. I used to tell those guys to take a look at that other guy and to count their blessings.

So now, I have to look at things like that. I can see where they are coming from, because I can get around, but I'm still complaining and moaning. But I guess as long as I'm complaining and moaning, things aren't that bad. It could be a hell of a lot worse, and it's probably going to get a lot worse. However, in the meantime, count your blessings. I've got a wonderful wife. I've got a wonderful daughter. I've got a son who's not crazy about this sort of stuff, but he does it. He helps take care of me. My daughter helps take care of me. They're not happy about it, but they do it.

I understand that I'm not exactly the easiest guy in the world to get along with, but I am still counting my blessings. It could be a whole lot worse. I am trying to sit down and accept things the way they are. This is something that is really hard to do sometimes, but you have to keep going. You have to. There is no alternative. I suggest having someone to vent and rant to, because talking about this helps me feel better.

I also got myself a service dog. She's not a real service dog, but she is a three-year-old puppy, and she curls up on the couch with me. We cuddle up, and that makes me feel a lot better. There is a song by Tom T. Hall called "Old Dogs, Children, and Watermelon Wine." In the song, he talks about watermelon wine and little children before they're too young to hate and how all dogs love you no matter what. Dogs give you that unconditional love. So I would recommend anyone to get themselves a pet. If you're old, get an older pet, like an older dog. They make you feel better, and they always give you unconditional love.

> **"I'm not exactly an angel; I never have been. I'm not the nicest guy in the world, but I don't think I deserve this."**

**Expert Comment:**

Patients with underlying psychological problems like PTSD, anxiety, or depression may get worse facing the stress of a new diagnosis, especially of an unpredictable disease like MG. Steroids can cause frank psychosis, but more commonly they cause personality changes toward anxiety and depression. This may complicate treatment, as many psychogenic symptoms may mimic MG symptoms, and patients expect them to improve with the treatment of MG; in fact, they may worsen.

Some patients may need to see a psychiatrist or a counselor to treat these disorders. Also, these patients may have a negative attitude toward treatment, and they may be poorly compliant with the prescribed medications. They tend to change the dosage on their own and to miss appointments. It is important to set their expectations from the start so that they will not be disappointed. Pets are often helpful as a part of psychotherapy.

> **"Steroids can cause frank psychosis."**

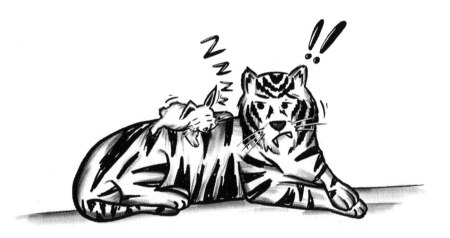

Roger... You're taking this lifestyle too far

# Case #44

## I Live a Normal Life

"I've made a lot of mistakes throughout my treatment that prolonged it… I stopped taking the medication during the tapering period…when you are young, you feel kind of invincible."

During the late summer of 2014, I began to experience drooping eyelids and double vision. I was particularly impacted by these occurrences while driving. The symptoms would come and go as I adjusted to overcome the more minor effects. As it got more prevalent, I realized something was wrong.

Over the next two to three months, I had appointments with my family doctor, my optometrist, and another eye specialist. I had scans for a brain tumor and a thymus gland tumor, both with negative results. At that point, I was referred to a neurologist who diagnosed me with myasthenia gravis.

To address the issue, I was prescribed 80 mg of prednisone per day. My symptoms were overcome within about two or three weeks, but I continued the initial recommended dosage for several months. Over the last five and a half years, we have continued to reduce the dosage. Twice, I have had minor recurrences of my symptoms, which we were able to control by increasing the dosage for a limited time. The current control dosage is 10 mg every other day.

During my treatment, I had a period of about two months when I had a loss of taste and minor difficulty swallowing; these went away without any additional medication. Also, early in my treatment, when my dosage of prednisone was high, I did not sleep as much and would awake after five to six hours with plenty of energy. That dissipated over time as my dosage decreased. Today, my MG is under control and does not impact my normal daily routine.

> *"Today, my MG is under control and does not impact my normal daily routine."*

**Expert Comment:**

Insomnia (lack of or reduced sleep) is common in MG, either due to depression or as a side effect of steroids. It is recommended that prednisone is taken in the morning. Sleep apnea, which can be worsened by steroids, is another cause of insomnia. Simple measures should be tried first, such as taking a warm shower, avoiding eating for four hours before bedtime, and weight loss. Over-the-counter diphenhydramine (Benadryl) 25 mg at bedtime is usually helpful. If not, the physician may prescribe medication for insomnia that does not interfere with MG or its medications.

> *"Insomnia in a myasthenic can have many causes."*

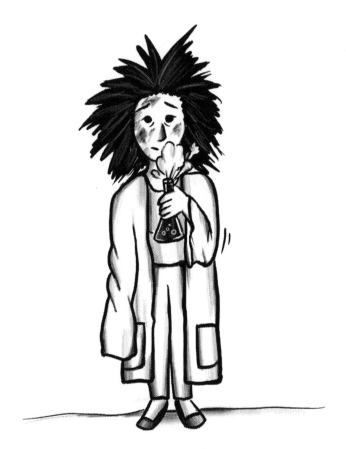

Trust your doctor

# Case #45

## Do Not Stop the Medicine on Your Own

I was diagnosed with myasthenia gravis in December of 2016, at the age of nineteen. I was fortunate in the fact that I was only diagnosed with ocular MG. I had always been proud of my eyesight. I was the only one in the family not wearing glasses, and when I was hit with the symptoms, I was just confused at what was going on. I started getting horrendous double vision and would have to tilt my head in a specific manner in order to get my eyes to line up.

I remember being called out on it a lot. My friends would ask me, "Why are you holding your head like that?" and I would have to explain.

I lived like that for nearly a month without really thinking about going to the doctor. A couple of weeks later, I had my annual optometry appointment. My optometrist was not sure what it was; originally, it was thought to be an extreme astigmatism, and I was prescribed glasses for it. But the optometrist also referred me to a specialist out of town.

The optometrist there spent nearly three hours with me and told me I would need an MRI because there was a possibility that it was a tumor. I remember seeing my mom's face when she heard that—very distraught and genuinely scared, processing what may come from this due to the fact that there is a family history of cancer.

I remember my parents talking about the fact that they had just switched our health insurance to one with a higher deductible and a lower premium, so they were going to have to pay a decent amount of the cost of testing. Thankfully, the MRI came back negative, and the institute referred me to my new doctor. I've been a patient there ever since.

One of the things I love about my new doctor is how straight to the point he was, giving me accurate information that I needed to know. I remember being quite relieved by my diagnosis. I mean, it sucks for sure, having this autoimmune disease where your body is literally fighting against itself, but with the potential of cancer on the table, this was the best I could have hoped for. I was immediately put onto a steroid treatment that would last for two years: a strong dose of prednisone every day for several months with an eventual tapering period.

As with all medication, there were pros and cons. The myasthenia was gone—no more double vision. The eyesight I had always been proud of was back, and I was happy with that. The side effects, though not life-threatening in any way, weren't fun to deal with. I had some extreme acne from which I still have some scars on my face, and some extreme weight gain that has been a struggle for me to lose. We're talking thirty pounds over the course of two years.

I've made a lot of mistakes throughout my treatment that prolonged it and caused my side effects to lengthen their time with me. Twice, I stopped taking the medication during the tapering period. Just a bad decision on my part, but when you are young, you feel kind of invincible. The symptoms of your disease go away, and you just think to yourself, *All right, it's done, I'm good now.* Both times, my symptoms came back, the double vision was back, and I was holding my head back in those specific ways, probably looking weird to most people. I would come back to my doctor, and he let me know that if I screwed this up again for the third time, I would have to find a different neurologist.

Since my last undertaking of the steroid treatment, I have nearly finished with my taper, and thankfully I am still experiencing no symptoms of MG. I am lucky that this has been only ocular for me. It has not hindered my ability to do physical activity or exercise, even though there has been a weight gain. In my life, I am still active; I just kind of eat more.

Myasthenia has been a pain for sure, but with doctors like my current doctor around, they really help you through this process. Even though it's not curable, they will treat it to the best of their ability. I full-heartedly thank him and the staff for doing everything they have done for me.

> ## *"I've made a lot of mistakes throughout my treatment that prolonged the suffering."*

**Expert Comment:**

Acne is a common side effect of steroids. Especially at a young age, it can be embarrassing. Fortunately, it goes away after the prednisone is lowered to an effective and safe maintenance dose, which is usually 10–20 mg every other day. Rarely, a dermatology consultation is needed to treat the acne.

Diplopia can force patients to tilt their head to unify the image. That is the case when one of the eye-moving muscles is affected, especially the superior oblique.

Some patients change the dose or stop the medication on their own when they get better. The risk of relapse is high, and to suppress the disease, one has to start high-dose prednisone again, as going one step back is usually not effective. Symptoms may take weeks to return after stopping the medicine. Poor compliance with medical orders may lead to a life-threatening relapse that may mandate artificial ventilation.

> ## *"Poor compliance with medical orders may lead to a life-threatening relapses."*

Doctor, did you get my message?

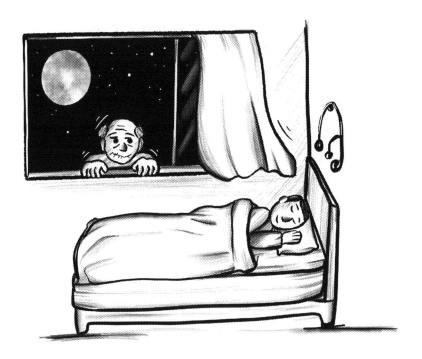

# Case #46

## BE SURE YOUR MG PHYSICIAN IS ACCESSIBLE

"My nature is to plan for the worst, but that also
forces me to look for an exit strategy to get past
whatever unresolved situation I face"

I am a seventy-nine-year-old man who lives in a small community about seventy-five miles from a major city. I was first diagnosed with myasthenia gravis in 2014. The symptoms I had were a drooping eyelid and slurred speech. Those symptoms resulted in my primary doctor thinking I was having a series of TIAs. It wasn't until I went to the stroke center in a large city that the diagnosis of MG was made.

Neither my wife nor I had ever heard of MG, so we really had no idea what our new journey would be. My interest is in warning new patients that many medical professionals do not have much experience with MG, and you must have an advocate who can help you manage the system if needed. As mentioned above, my primary physician attributed my MG symptoms to possible stroke symptoms. It took a couple of days before a physician at a different hospital linked my symptoms to other autoimmune illnesses. I have vitiligo and diabetes; no one had mentioned possible MG.

Shortly after the diagnosis, I was on a car trip when my symptoms became worse. We called my neurologist and tried to get a prescription for Mestinon from three pharmacies on our route. None of them had it in stock. Fortunately, the fourth pharmacy we contacted had the medication.

In July 2015, my swallowing became so difficult that I went to our local hospital emergency room. My wife could not get the ER physician to acknowledge that I was in a dangerous condition. He eventually called my physician, who recognized that I was in an MG crisis. I was sent by Life Flight helicopter to a major city for treatment with IVIG. I was intubated for about a week and ended up spending over three weeks in the hospital.

A few weeks after my discharge, I had to go to an ER out of town. My swallowing and breathing were compromised. The ER triage nurse said my O2 sat was 98 percent, so there was nothing wrong with my breathing. She did not know that a nonfunctioning diaphragm could be the problem. The ER physician spoke with my doctor and was told to administer Mestinon in IV form. The hospital did not have it, so my own liquid Mestinon, which I carry at all times, was given to me by way of an NG tube.

When the physician was first told I had MG, he started googling it on his phone as we talked to my current doctor, who has treated me with prednisone and azathioprine before. Prednisone has many side effects that are difficult to live with. Over a long period of time, the prednisone dosage has been reduced until I am on a maintenance dosage that appears to be working well. I do not toy with my medications in any way, fearing I will cause another crisis. The only relapse I've had was when the prednisone was reduced too much.

The levels of prednisone and azathioprine have now put me into a stable balance. We always carry a list of medications to avoid. When I was recently diagnosed with pneumonia, the list came in handy regarding which antibiotics to avoid. My doctor's office was contacted before the antibiotics were called into the pharmacy.

My daily life with MG seems to be most affected by fatigue and muscle weakness. Just getting up in the morning, taking my meds, and showering is exhausting. I often go back to bed for a while to regain my strength. Walking long distances and standing still for long periods are particularly challenging. When we travel by plane, I always use wheelchair assistance in the airport.

I would like to think that more physicians, nurses, and ancillary personnel will be more knowledgeable of myasthenia gravis, but until that is the case, every patient and caregiver needs to be ready to help educate them. Most importantly, be sure your MG physician is accessible.

> *"The only relapse I've had was when the prednisone was reduced too much."*

**Expert Comment:**

Symptoms of MG may present acutely and or progress quickly, leading to the wrong diagnosis of stroke or transient ischemic attack. Because MG is not common while stroke is, the latter is more commonly thought of as a diagnosis to explain sudden slurring of speech, impairment of swallowing, double vision, etc.

Shortness of breath may progress to a point where the patient cannot maintain safe breathing, and intubation and artificial ventilation is the only way to save life. Fortunately, people rarely die from MG due to the advancement and availability of treatment modalities such as plasma exchange and IVIG. However, patients with multiple medical problems like cancer, renal failure, COPD, uncontrolled diabetes, and hypertension may not be able to tolerate the burden of an MG crisis.

It is important for treating physicians to make themselves available all the time to their patients. Very often, the covering on-call physician does not have access to the medical records and is not familiar with the specific patient condition; therefore, if possible, treating physicians should take the first call even if they are out of town so that they can provide the best advice.

> *"It is important for treating physicians to make themselves available all the time to their patients."*

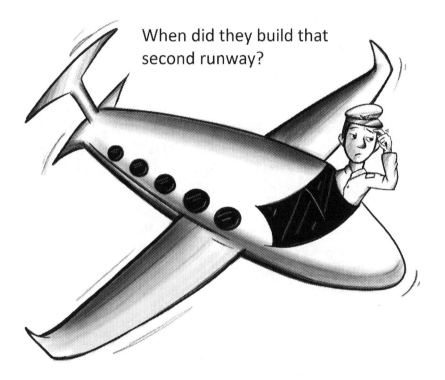

# Case #47

## A Pilot with Diplopia

"Patients with personal or family history of other autoimmune disease – such as type one diabetes mellitus—are at a higher risk of developing MG, which is also an autoimmune disease."

A brief background biography: I was born in 1965. My only sibling, a brother, was born in 1970, after which my mother was diagnosed with rheumatoid arthritis. She suffered pain and gradual joint deterioration for thirty years and passed away at age fifty-seven after hospitalization for a relatively innocuous illness. My first child, born in 1995, was diagnosed with autoimmune hepatitis in 1999 and received a liver transplant in 2008; she is doing quite well today. In 2009, I was diagnosed with type 2 diabetes (DM) and have been able to control it without insulin. My job as a pilot does not allow the use of insulin, per the FAA.

I am providing my family's health history because I have always wondered if there was any connection between the autoimmune conditions my mother, myself (myasthenia gravis), and my daughter have encountered. The professionals I have asked over the years have all assured me they are unrelated, but I still find the situation curious.

In my youth, I was on the chunkier side, but I was pretty active and enjoyed physical activity. In high school, I played team sports and eventually became quite fit. I was accepted to the US Naval Academy, which led to fourteen years in the navy, requiring me to maintain a high level of fitness. When I separated from the navy in 1996, I was in very good health.

Since 1996, I have worked as a pilot for UPS, flying large aircraft. The nature of UPS's operation is mostly overnight duty, which obviously contributes to fatigue and a less-than-optimal immune system. I went through periods of gaining weight followed by periods of consistent exercise. I will say that the added stress of a child living with liver disease leading to a transplant contributed to poorer overall health.

Now to MG: After ten or so years of maintaining control of the DM, I was in a pretty good place overall. I was probably on the down cycle of physical fitness and maybe ten pounds overweight. Typically, I work week-on/week-off, meaning overnight flying Monday through Friday one week then really about nine days off. After twenty years, I have become accustomed to dealing with the sleep flip-flops relatively well.

In early July 2017, after my last overnight work period, I was driving home from the airport and felt very sleepy. My left eyelid felt heavy. Assuming I was just very tired, I got home and slept. Everything seemed relatively normal after getting rest. During that week off, I did start to feel like my left eye was intermittently just a little droopy, but not so much as to obscure my vision. My wife would occasionally notice the slight droop.

The following Friday, I worked overnight, and during the weekend layover the left eyelid became heavy again. I forced myself to get lots of sleep, but I was beginning to believe something else was going on. Very well rested on Monday night (July 10), on the first flight into our base, I was unable to keep my left eye open. After landing, I reported sick and caught a ride home. I was pretty scared. I even remember thinking during the last landing, *Is this the last flight of my career?*

> **"I was pretty scared. I even remember thinking during the last landing, Is this the last flight of my career?"**

The next morning, July 11, I broke the news to my wife, who scheduled an appointment with the ophthalmologist for the next day. After getting past my denial, I started researching everything about ptosis (droopy eyelid), its causes, and its treatment. I remember MG being one cause, but that sounded like something rare, so I looked to other causes.

I started researching surgeries or special glasses to prop the eyelid open based on what I was reading. My nature is to plan for the worst, but that also forces me to look for an exit strategy to get past whatever unresolved situation I face. Surgery seemed extreme, so I pictured myself with the special eyeglasses—a little unusual, but not the worst thing.

The next day's appointment, on July 12, wasn't conclusive, but the doctor believed it was myasthenia gravis and referred me to a neuro-ophthalmologist. Fortunately, I was able to get an appointment two days later.

Now I finally gave in and did some research on MG. My memory of how I felt while reading was that I had a very rare disease that wasn't necessarily life-threatening but was certainly life-changing. I wasn't sure what the treatment might entail, but I assumed it might disqualify me from flying. I was already dealing with special circumstances with the FAA due to my DM. With so many questions and so little information, my career seemed in jeopardy.

On the fourteenth, I had an exhaustive (literally) exam with my neuro-ophthalmologist, including eye exercises that exacerbated the droopy eyelid. In the end, the doctor diagnosed the MG, which was confirmed by antibody blood tests. Obviously, MG was not the doctor's specialty. I remember she tried to give me some ideas of treatment, but my overall fear for my future remained. She referred me to an MG specialist, and fortunately, I was able to get an appointment two weeks later.

The two-week wait was reasonable, but of course, I was still very down about my outlook. I began to think about a career change, although that seemed daunting. On a positive note, I started a daily exercise routine, which distracted me from my worries and made me feel better. Also, my job did have a pretty good disability program. At that point, I had enough sick time to cover three to four months of full pay. Should I go beyond that, the program paid about two-thirds pay for two years. I was definitely stressed about our financial situation, but I knew we had some time until it would become more difficult.

Finally, August 1 came, and I had my first appointment with the MG specialist. Going into the appointment, my wife and I were quite anxious due to our lack of knowledge. My overall memory of the visit is the doctor telling us, "This is quite treatable, and we'll get you back to normal." For whatever reason—maybe I was afraid to research too deeply on the internet or because it was my nature to prepare for the worst—I hadn't expected such an optimistic prognosis. Of course, the treatment to get me back to work right away was easier said than done, but I now had an exit strategy that I could feel good about.

My doctor answered my many questions patiently, and I left the appointment feeling better than I had since that last flight. A subsequent thyroid scan was negative—which reminds me to mention I also have hypothyroidism treated with Synthroid. That was diagnosed in 2009 and has remained stable.

To initially treat the ptosis, I was prescribed pyridostigmine bromide. I found that it was somewhat effective in decreasing the droopy eyelid, although it did not always work. I tried it during the first week or so after my initial visit. The main treatment was a high dose of prednisone (80 mg). The doctor predicted it would kick in after about a week. Sure enough, a week later, the left eye was no longer sagging. At that point, I discontinued the pyridostigmine.

The course of steroids called for a high dosage for six weeks followed by a gradual four- to five-month taper. To be honest, my experience with 80 mg prednisone daily was not all that bad. I had a lot of energy (I was up every day early making breakfast), continued my daily exercise, and focused on many projects around the house. I understand there are hazards of long-term use of steroids. I have been taking calcium to counter the effects of steroid use.

Because of the large steroid doses, I needed to start supplementing my DM care with long- and short-acting insulin to help with my A1C level. Since I was not cleared to fly anyway, this was acceptable for now. My endocrinologist felt confident that I would not become reliant on insulin when the prednisone level was reduced to a much lower maintenance dose. Still, this added slightly to the concern of my future flying.

It was during these months of waiting to wean off the steroid levels that I was able to see a path back to work. Contrary to my normal process, I told myself, *This is going to work. Yes, there are some unknowns about how to get cleared by the FAA, but it will work out.* I found a little bit of inner peace during that time, knowing I couldn't change the prescribed regimen, so I enjoyed being at home for a while.

I also looked for silver linings. My younger two children were a sophomore and a senior in high school. I got to spend much more time with them and attend all of their activities. I really don't think I have ever experienced any noticeable side effects from any of the medications for MG. I dutifully followed the doctors tapering schedule in hopes of being at an FAA-approved level of prednisone in January 2018.

> *"Because of the large steroid doses, I needed to start supplementing my DM care with long- and short-acting insulin."*

Unfortunately, in late December, I began to realize I was feeling a little different. I was a little more tired, but I thought it was from the reduction in energy from the prednisone. Then in January, my right eyelid started to droop. I was devastated. Fortunately, my doctor was able to see me right away. Once again, he was confident I would be able to recover. Plan A had been steroids. Plan B now was the addition of azathioprine. Interestingly enough, I was familiar with azathioprine, since my daughter had been taking it post-transplant.

Of course, I had to start a new course of high-dose steroids followed by a taper. This was a disappointment and put me in a month or so of depression. The good news was that although the ptosis took a little longer to resolve (ten to fourteen days), it has been gone for over two years now. I ended up being at home the whole school year, which allowed for a lot of quality time with the family.

The last real hurdle was getting clearance from the FAA. Commercial pilots are required to pass an FAA physical every six months (every twelve months if under forty) called a medical certificate. Many medical conditions allow for qualification, but only after further documentation and review by the FAA resulting in a special issuance (SI). I had been able to maintain an SI certificate for my DM since my diagnosis in 2009.

My pilot union retains a medical advisor to help with the SI process. This doctor had helped me over the years with the DM SI, so I contacted him soon after my diagnosis. He was not familiar with any pilots with an MG SI, but he was optimistic about the potential for approval. The fact that he worked for a major airline for many years and now advises several pilot groups (thousands of pilots!) speaks to the rare nature of MG.

Long story short, in June of 2018, I was finally stable—the MG specialist tells me I'm in remission—and on a dose of prednisone that is acceptable to the FAA. The process took longer than I had hoped. Status reports from several doctors, lab reports, and eye exams were submitted. Follow-ups with more details were requested. All this time, I remained positive if somewhat impatient.

Finally, in October 2018, I received the SI for MG and passed my physical. A couple of weeks later, I was back in training, and by January 2019, I was back to work full time.

> *"Finally, I was back in training, and by January 2019, I was back to work full time as a pilot."*

**Expert Comment:**

Diplopia is inconvenient to everyone but dangerous to some professionals, such as truck drivers and pilots. No one would feel safe in an airplane if the pilot has droopy eyelids and double vision. Before releasing a pilot back to work, a longer remission period is needed than for other professions. Six months of remission would be reasonable. The pilot should stop flying with even a hint of recurrence of the symptoms. Medications used for MG are not sedating and do not cause sleepiness.

Patients with personal or family history of other autoimmune diseases—such as type one diabetes mellitus, thyroid disease, rheumatoid arthritis, and multiple sclerosis—are at a higher risk of developing MG, which is also an autoimmune disease. Thyroid disorders can cause symptoms similar to MG or can exacerbate MG. Exophthalmos (bulging of the eyes) is a feature of excessive thyroid function that leads to thickening of the eye-moving muscles. Diplopia is common, but instead of droopy eyelids, they get lid retraction, where the eyes are open wider than normal. Thyroid enlargement (goiter) can cause swallowing difficulty like MG. Fatigue, shortness of breath, and leg weakness are common to both. It takes an expert to treat a patient who carries the diagnosis of both.

> *"Diplopia is inconvenient to everyone but dangerous to some professionals, such as truck drivers and pilots."*

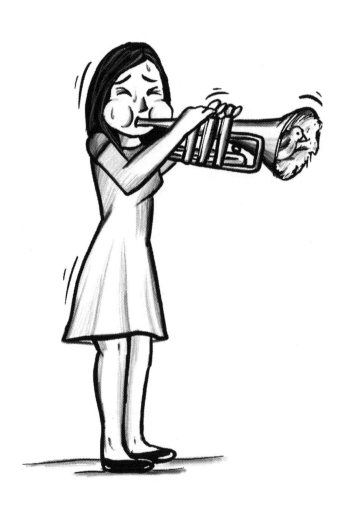

# Case #48

## I Could Not Play the Trumpet Anymore

"Taking the medication was difficult. I thought the cure was going to kill me there for a while; that's how bad I felt."

My story begins in 1983, about thirty-six years ago, when I was sixteen. My earliest symptoms happened when I was playing in my high school's marching band. I used to play the trumpet, and there were times when I couldn't get my lips tight enough to blow through the mouthpiece. I was struggling, so I decided to change instruments and switched to the baritone. I thought that the bigger mouthpiece on the baritone would make it easier to blow. However, that was not the case, and I still had difficulty. I ended up quitting band my senior year of high school.

My older sister noticed that on my sixteenth birthday, I had a hard time blowing out the candles on my cake. I've never had any issues breathing. In high school, I ran four years of track, running the half-mile, one mile, two mile, and the two-mile relay. I also ran three years of cross-country.

When I first went to the doctor, they thought it was some kind of allergy, so they put me on allergy medication. However, that didn't work, so I was sent to the children's hospital. They did a swallow test and couldn't find anything wrong. I also went to a speech therapist, and again, that didn't help.

Years went by. I got married, had four children, and moved to a different state. By 1994, my doctor requested a muscle biopsy on my arm.

But once again, nothing was found, because everything from my neck down was fine. Doctors still didn't know what was wrong, and there was still no treatment.

My condition was worsening, and it was getting more difficult to talk, eat, and swallow. When I talk, I have to slow it down so people can understand me. The people who are around me a lot and know me well can understand me. A lot of the time, my family, my friends, or my kids would be my translators. To this day, sometimes they still are.

As for eating, I have always been a slow eater. I guess that has been a good thing. I just have to chew my food more. I've never been one to inhale my food, so to speak.

Taking any kind of medicine has always been a battle for me. First of all, I don't like to take medications. Any pills I take have to be chewable or small enough to swallow, because I can't take horse-sized pills. If it's a pill I have to swallow, I have to line it up in my throat just right, and I have to chase it down with milk or something hot, like coffee or tea. Otherwise, the pill will get stuck in my throat, and it's very difficult to get it unstuck.

I wasn't diagnosed with myasthenia gravis until 2001. I was prescribed 60 mg of pyridostigmine three times a day. I also had a CT scan on my thymus gland. They said my thymus gland was fine and nothing else was done. I took that pill for nineteen years.

This brings us to the present. My then-doctor referred me to an MG specialist. I started seeing this specialist in February of 2019. The specialist said that I had the worst case of MG that he had ever seen.

I am now taking 20 mg of prednisone, one tablet every other day. I am also taking 50 mg of azathioprine, one tablet three times a day. On November 5, 2019, I had my thymus gland taken out. They say it takes about a year to see any results, so we shall see. I think that I am getting better. I can suck through a straw again. I have to use the side of my mouth, but I can do it. I know the more rest I get, the better I sound. Some days are better than others, but I do think that I'm getting better.

> **"The specialist said that I had the worst case of MG that he had ever seen."**

**Expert Comment:**

Weakness of the facial muscles is not unusual in MG, and sometimes it becomes the most disabling feature. Patients cannot blow their lips to kiss or to inflate a balloon or to play a trumpet. This can be life-changing if the patient happens to play trumpet for living. Also, weak lips causes slurring of speech and difficulty pronouncing the labial sounds like *B*, *M*, *P*, and *V*. With time, the configuration of the lips may become deformed due to chronic weakness, and the mouth will become crooked. This is usually compounded by weakness of the tongue.

Swallowing problems may prevent ingestion of medications, which will make MG worse. These patients may benefit from changing the tablets to solutions or rarely injections. If the disease is that severe, it may be useful to treat with IVIG in order to restore swallowing function, then start the oral medications.

Pyridostigmine (Mestinon) is used to treat the symptoms. It does not change the course of the disease and does not address the underlying autoimmune process. If it does not work, steroids should be seriously considered to avoid long-term complications. When the disease remains ineffectively treated for a long time, some of the weak muscles become weak permanently, and even aggressive treatment will do little.

> *"If the disease is that severe, it may be useful to treat with IVIG in order to restore swallowing function, then start the oral medications."*

Your surgery is in one hour

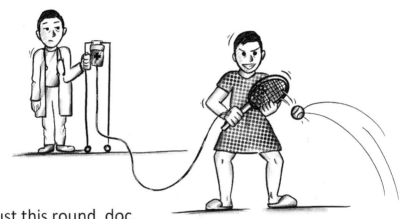

Just this round, doc.

# Case #49

## Keep Doing Things As You're Able

*"First, I would like to start off saying that myasthenia gravis is not a death sentence."*

The first symptom I experienced was one day, all of a sudden, I could not see well. I have had dry macular degeneration for years, so I go to the ophthalmologist regularly. Two weeks before I started to experience the sudden vision problems, I was put on a vitamin regimen for my macular degeneration. Two weeks later, I couldn't read, I couldn't see the TV, and I was having trouble driving. So I went ahead and called my ophthalmologist to make an appointment, because I thought my macular degeneration had worsened or something.

When I went in to see the ophthalmologist, he said it might be something else, and he referred me to my general practitioner. My general practitioner began running tests, and in fact, one of the tests he sent off to California. That test took a few weeks to get back, maybe three to four weeks, and when it came back, it came back positive for myasthenia gravis. In total, it took about six weeks to finally be diagnosed with MG.

When I first heard the diagnosis, I was very, very concerned. I'd heard of the disease before, and I knew that it affected the eyes. The doctor says it does not affect the acuity of your eyes. But otherwise, my eyes have just degenerated rapidly since the diagnosis, and I don't think it has anything to do with MG. It just has to do with the fact that my eyes are getting worse.

After my diagnosis, my general practitioner communicated with my ophthalmologist, and he's the one who made the appointment for me with a specialist in the MG field. He told me that this doctor was an expert in this disease. So very shortly after, within two weeks, I went to see the specialist.

Upon seeing my MG specialist, I was stressed. I was very stressed, because I did not know what to expect. I did not know if my eyesight would improve. As soon as I went into the appointment, the doctor gave me some information on what to expect with the disease. After talking with him, I told him, "I'm in love."

He just laughed and asked, "Why?"

I said, "Well, because you gave me hope."

That first appointment, he immediately started me on a heavy dose of prednisone, every day. Although my eyesight got better as soon as I started the prednisone, I was feeling horrible, and I could not function. I did not feel well. I lost my appetite, and I didn't want to eat. All I did was mostly sit at home.

I'd never taken a steroid like that before, and I was not used to it. Taking the medication was difficult. I thought the cure was going to kill me there for a while; that's how bad I felt. Luckily, both of my daughters live within a half mile of my house—so close in fact that I can see their house from my house. They were always very attentive and made sure that I was okay and taken care of.

Anyway, the doctor reduced the dosage slowly. I was taking 70 mg for a period of time, and then he reduced it to 60 mg, and I took that for months; then he reduced it to 40 mg. He brought me down very slowly, and of course, the lower the dosage got, the better I felt. He brought me down to 15 mg of prednisone, which I was taking every other day.

To make sure I followed the plans exactly, the doctor gave me a day-by-day chart to mark off each day I took the medication so that I would not forget. There wasn't any way I was going to forget, but it was helpful.

There was a time I did have a setback in my myasthenia. It was before one of my appointments with the doctor. My neck began to hurt, and I thought that I had hurt my neck when I was mowing the grass. I live in the country, so I have a lot of grass to mow. I've always fallen in holes and stuff, but all of a sudden my neck was really sore, and it was really bothering me. I couldn't even hold my head up. I had to mentally and physically pick my head up. If I didn't try to pick it up, I was just looking at the floor all the time.

I finally went to my doctor's appointment, and as soon as I told him my neck was killing me, he immediately put me back on a heavier dose of 60 mg a day for a short while. This time, he brought me down a lot faster. So as of today, I've been taking 20 mg every other day for the past three months or even longer. I was told to stay on 20 mg every other day until I saw him again, but I haven't seen him yet due to the coronavirus. To this day, I am not sure what exactly caused me to have a relapse.

I used to think MG would only affect me from the shoulders up. However, I started having other problems, and my doctor said MG can affect your joints and your muscles. Right now, I'm having a real problem with my left hip, and my doctor suggested that I check with a bone and joint doctor, so I did. The doctor believed it was bursitis and prescribed therapy. I don't think the therapy helped much, and I don't know what's causing the problem. I can walk, but I have to use a cane, because without it, my legs would give out and I would fall. The hip problem could be due to a combination of things.

I have noticed that my ability to do some physical activity is slowed by MG. It's not hard to do therapy. In fact, I felt much better after therapy, but we had to stop because of this virus. But anyways, I noticed I felt better. I could walk better, even though I still needed to use my cane; I could still walk. I noticed the days I take prednisone, I do better. It's not much, but it's better.

The problem has not gone away, but thankfully, I have not fallen yet. I have a big fear that I will fall and break a bone, but so far that has not happened. The days I do not take prednisone, it's much harder to walk, and it is painful. It's not great pain, but you feel it.

I cannot work on my house like I used to—like I can't clean out a cabinet or my closets. However, I can do the housework, but I need to do it carefully, like mopping the floors, the laundry, and cooking. I just can't work in my yard. I am not sure if my fatigue is from the MG, but I know I do not have any energy.

I do read a lot and just do quiet things. I work at something for an hour, and I sit an hour, work for an hour and sit an hour. I have always been very active, and I'm noticing I sleep more. Sometimes I sleep nine hours. For me, that is very unusual.

Also, my eyesight is to the point where I don't drive. My daughters or my sons-in-law have to take me everywhere. So I stay at home, and that's one thing I hate—the fact that I can't drive anymore. I mean, I could, but they are afraid for me to. I see much better the days I take prednisone. Normally, about four o'clock in the afternoon, my sight clears up, and it is sharper. It is weird. It just affects you in the weirdest ways.

Myasthenia gravis did affect me psychologically a bit, because it changed the appearance of my face. The prednisone caused me to have a round-looking face, and now my eyes are always puffy. I also think it has made me look a little older. I am currently eighty-three, so I should be looking older anyway, but I feel like I look older than I should. I don't look quite the same as I did before all this started about two or three years ago.

The change in my face and my hip pain are the only things I'm dealing with right now. The round face started to go away when we started tapering down the medication, but it is still there a little bit. It just changes your appearance so much, and at this point, I didn't want to look any worse than I did. Meeting people and going to church was different now, because I was not wanting to be as social as I normally would be. People were not making too many remarks about it, but it was distressing.

One thing that helped me a lot, because of my age, was that the doctor looked at me and said, "You're not going to die from this." So that was a comfort. This disease is just something I'm going to have to deal with for the rest of my life, because the doctor told me I would be taking steroids to keep the symptoms under control. If I could still walk well and do the things I've always done and need to do around the house and for myself, then I feel like I could handle the MG better.

The thing that helped me the most was the encouragement from the doctor. He was telling me that I can do this, and I'm going to be okay. It is not a life-threatening disease—it is just something we have to deal with. I think that was the most important thing that helped me to accept what was happening.

My eyes have deteriorated to the point where I have to use a magnifying glass to read the newspaper or anything except a Kindle, where you can change the size of the print. If you're diagnosed with MG, the most important thing is just to follow the doctor's instructions to the letter. I also think the doctor is not just concerned with the disease he is treating, he is also concerned with the person. He wants to know if you're okay, and I am okay. I'm dealing with it. I have strong support from friends and from my family. That's important too.

Keeping up your social life is important. Make sure to keep seeing people. Keep going places, and keep doing things as you're able.

> *"The thing that helped me the most was the encouragement from the doctor."*

**Expert Comment:**

MG does not cause a loss of visual acuity. It is important to have an ophthalmological examination in these cases to rule out causes of loss of vision, such as stroke, cataract, glaucoma, and macular degeneration. Steroids may produce or worsen cataracts and glaucoma. The only way MG can occlude vision is by causing complete droopiness of the eyelids.

There are certain symptoms that should raise the possibility of another or concomitant diagnosis; those include loss of vision, numbness or tingling, severe pain behind the eyes, severe headache, loss of strength on one side of the body, and loss of bladder control. Steroids may worsen diabetes and hypertension and may accelerate the occurrence of stroke and vascular blindness.

> *"MG does not cause a loss of visual acuity."*

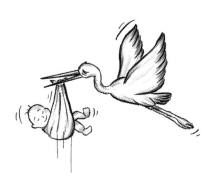

That MG bird brought the
wrong species again

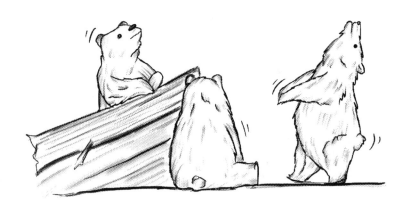

# Case #50

## PREGNANT AND COPING WITH MYASTHENIA GRAVIS

First, I would like to start off saying that myasthenia gravis is not a death sentence. I was officially diagnosed with MG at the age of twenty-seven, after having my third baby. You can imagine my anxiety levels during this joyous time. I had been experiencing mild symptoms since I was twenty-one years old, after having my second child. My symptoms presented as weakness in my arms whenever I was lifting something. I would also have weakness in my legs walking or going up and down stairs. Mild exercise became unbearable, as it felt like I couldn't control my body anymore. In the back of my mind, I just thought my body really hated me.

I began searching my symptoms online, and everything pointed to anemia. I went to see my primary-care doctor, who just brushed it under the table. I went on six more years with these symptoms. My husband and I decided we wanted to have another child in 2012, and I became pregnant. During pregnancy, all my symptoms just vanished, and I felt like myself again.

I gave birth to a healthy baby boy; he experienced no complications, and neither did I. Everything was going great post-pregnancy for the first three months. I had no weakness, and I thought, *Man, this is the life.* I didn't realize that I was in for the shock of my life.

Four months post-pregnancy, my symptoms returned with a vengeance, this time affecting my vision first. I had a droopy eye that I could barely see out of, which made driving extremely difficult. Then I developed slurred speech. I could barely talk, eat, or swallow. I eventually lost forty pounds over the course of two weeks. Since I was unable to chew food, I resorted to drinking smoothies and eating mashed potatoes.

The weakness in my arms returned, and now it affected my hands. I was unable to hold my baby or perform any hygiene care alone. I'd finally had enough and went to the emergency room, but all my labs and scans came back normal. The ER doctor told me that he could see increased secretions on my scan and referred me to an ENT doctor.

I finally saw the ENT, and he performed an in-office scope and saw pooling of secretions around my voice box. He then referred me to a neurologist. Before I could see the neurologist, my symptoms got worse. While walking to the car, my legs collapsed from under me. I was lying on the ground with my body so limp, I was unable to lift myself from the ground to reach my phone. I finally got the phone and called my husband to pick me up off the ground.

That day, he called the neurologist to explain what had happened and that I needed an appointment immediately. I finally was seen three days later and was officially diagnosed with myasthenia gravis. My neurologist said that I was the worst case she had seen. I was just grateful to finally know what was slowly destroying my daily life.

Being diagnosed with MG scared me at first until I understood that I could still live a normal life with medications and treatment. I was hospitalized for four days receiving IVIG treatments until I was able to swallow without aspirating. I didn't experience any side effects from IVIG treatments, but I could feel the sudden remission of my symptoms.

I then was placed on prednisone and pyridostigmine. The side effects of prednisone pushed me to gain twenty-five pounds in a week, whereas with the pyridostigmine, I would have diarrhea. The medications helped me get back to normal. The prednisone was eventually changed due to the rapid weight gain. I was then started on azathioprine, and this was a potent drug, as it could increase your chances of developing skin cancer. I limited the amount of time I spent outside. I had to come in for monthly labs to monitor my blood levels.

I followed my plan strictly and felt better every day I was on medication. If I experienced any symptoms, I would just sit down and rest. If I exerted myself too much, then I might develop some mild weakness. I was able to incorporate mild exercise back into my routine at least as much as I could tolerate.

> **"Being diagnosed with MG scared me at first
> until I understood that I could still live a
> normal life with medications and treatment."**

Post hospital admission, I have not experienced any relapses due to following my treatment regimen. I do experience diplopia from time to time. I was prescribed glasses, and it helps me out a lot, especially if I need to drive.

Something that has helped me through this journey is understanding my diagnosis. I would limit the amount of time in the sun because it could cause muscle weakness. I would go out early in the day to prevent over-exhaustion. Always keep a medical bracelet with your diagnosis, because there are medications and vaccines that we are not to take.

Don't let this diagnosis take over your life. Many people thought because I was so young that I would fall into a depression, and I did the exact opposite. I became a registered nurse, and I'm currently working on my MSN in family nurse practitioner.

**Expert Comment:**

MG may exacerbate during pregnancy or within a few weeks after delivery. Pregnant myasthenics should be under the care of a high-risk obstetrician. After delivery, the baby may not be able to breathe due to transfer of antibodies from the mother. This is usually a transient condition, but it is vital that it is treated early to prevent respiratory compromise.

MG relapses are not predictable, and one has to make available all the necessary measures and phone numbers in the house, office, and car.

Steroids and pyridostigmine are not contraindicated during pregnancy, but steroid-sparing agents such as azathioprine and methotrexate should be avoided during childbearing age because they may have an ill effect on the baby (teratogenic).

Printed in the United States
By Bookmasters